He's Not Autistic, But...

He's Not Autistic, But...

How We Pulled Our Son
From the Mouth of the Abyss

Tenna Merchent, M.H.

Joyous Messenger, Inc.
NOBLESVILLE, INDIANA

First printing 2007

ISBN 978-1-933697-00-0
LCCN 2006931387

**ATTENTION CORPORATIONS, UNIVERSITIES, COLLEGES,
AND PROFESSIONAL ORGANIZATIONS**: Quantity discounts are available
on bulk purchases of this book for educational, gift purposes, or as premiums.
Special books or book excerpts can also be created to fit specific needs.
For information, please contact Joyous Messenger, Inc.,
12160 E. 216th St., Noblesville, IN 46062.

Here's What People Are Saying About:

He's Not Autistic, But...

"I deeply admire the courage and determination of Tenna Merchent, who exerted great efforts and left no stone unturned to find a cure for her sick little boy. I have personally experienced how devastating autism can be to a family, and while her son was ultimately not afflicted with autism, I can relate with her endless journey to find a cure to end his suffering. After two years of attempting every traditional and alternative treatment for Clay, Tenna finally came across someone who understood her son's illness and provided a responsible treatment method. It was a painful journey, but thankfully, ended like a fairy-tale."

—Congressman Dan Burton [R-IN-05]

"Journey with the author as she slowly but surely learns that her pre-autistic baby was damaged by vaccines. Merchent's awakening—and her son's recovery—evolve from a complete acceptance of her doctors' advice, to doubts about conventional medicine, culminating with extreme gratitude at discovering the extraordinary benefits of alternative remedies. A true testament to the power of a mother's love to save her ailing child from modern healthcare."

—Neil Z. Miller
Author, *Vaccines: Are They Really Safe and Effective?*
Director, *Thinktwice Global Vaccine Institute*

"Tenna Merchent has written a compelling and heartwarming story about how she saved her son, Clay, from getting regressive autism. In the story she mentions the MMR vaccine that could have launched Clay into regressive autism. She mentions how she used natural therapies to help Clay and herself. Our family and others have seen the devastation the MMR vaccine had on our children."

—Raymond Gallup
Founder, *The Autism Autoimmunity Project*

"My father is a physician so I was much more accustomed to 'traditional' methods of treatment but Tenna's book was inspirational! When faced with a chronic illness or what seems like a hopeless situation, this book has given me just that—hope."
—Deb Castino
F.C. Tucker Company, Inc.
President's Club

"This book has given me a sense of relief that someone else has gone through what I have and come out of it with a happy and healthy child. It also began my journey into alternative medicines, doctors, and diets. I take my time making decisions that are best for my children rather than going forth with anything a conventional M.D. might recommend (especially if it involves just treating the symptoms with any drug, prescription or over the counter). I research and explore all possible options and I have learned how to pay attention to the 'whole child'; meaning not only my children's physical signs of discomfort, but the emotional and behavioral ones too. Everything is connected; and so far, everything has been treatable through diet and holistic avenues. I truly believe that the outcome would have been very different if this book had not started me down the path toward health."
—Nicki di Filippo
Computer Teacher
John Winthrop Middle School

TABLE OF CONTENTS

DEDICATION

This book is dedicated to my mother, Donta Roney. Without her help and guidance, we would never have found the cure to Clay's illness or to mine.

Unfortunately, we found our cure just a month before Mom died. Mom had been diagnosed with cancer in 1999 and was treated with chemotherapy and radiation. The treatment was worse than the disease. The last three years of her life were filled with pain, surgeries, and complications the treatment set in motion. I know Mom had a yeast overgrowth, and I suspect yeast and aluminum were the underlying cause of her illness— not cancer. She wasn't able to save herself; luckily, she saved us.

IN THANKS

Thank you, God, for giving me a story to write. If my son had not recovered there would be no story. Thank You for saving my son and my family. We were standing on a cliff overlooking autism; one more step and we would have fallen in. Divine intervention prevented us from taking that final step. I thank You so much for sparing us. You then brought him all the way back when you released the aluminum, baby shots, and parasites from his body. Thank You for giving me a healthy and happy son. You further blessed us by healing me, and giving me the gift of fertility, conception, and another healthy baby boy. You have been so generous to my family; I pray I am always grateful for these miraculous gifts.

Thank you, Master Herbalist. Without your intervention, we might never have found the cure to Clay's illness or mine. Thank you for all the sacrifices you and your family have made to help families like mine. Thank you also for allowing me to study with you. Your vast knowledge is a treasure, and I hope to share some of it with others through this book.

Thank you, Clay, for recovering. I am sorry the first two years of your life were so miserable. I'm sorry I passed my illness (aluminum) on to you, and I'm so sorry I let them give you those shots. I pray you can forgive me. Thank you for becoming the healthy, charming, bright, and fun little boy you are today.

Thank you, Mike (my husband), for supporting me as I searched for a cure. I know it was hard. I went down a lot of paths that turned out to be dead ends before we found the answer. Thank you for supporting me as I changed our lifestyle. Originally it was an effort to get healthy, then it became important to *support* our health. Thank you for all the nights you did the herbal combination W-W (an herbal combination for parasites) with Clay, and thank you for choking it down yourself. It's important our whole family be healthy.

Thank you, Barbra Dillenger. You have been so supportive and insightful. Your counseling and coaching as I faced different issues in each stage of this book were invaluable. Thank you for helping me to understand the law of noninterference, which is why we can't help people if they don't want help. You helped me realize how important it was to help others benefit from our experiences. Many of our conversations are reflected in this book; your footprints are all over it.

Thank you, Katherine Lehman. You were my first teacher in the healing art of releasing. Thank you for sharing your knowledge and time, and for filling in the blanks for me. Thank you for your friendship, guidance, and knowledge. Thank you for coaching me as I looked for additional cures for my family and friends. I couldn't have done this without you.

An Important Message to the Reader

This book is an account of my own experiences in seeking treatment for my son's physical ailments. As you will soon see, I was heartbroken by the unsuccessful results when I sought treatment from physicians and followed their advice in using conventional medicines. For that reason—and only after a great deal of research, study, and reflection—I made the decision to try prayer and various forms of alternative healing in place of conventional medicine. I did so out of my earnest belief in the power of prayer, and I believe that my son was able to regain his good health through these efforts.

As I have written elsewhere in this book, science isn't always the answer. Science has an important role in the world, but this type of healing works with the mystery, power, and beauty of nature of which we are a part and which our technologically oriented society tends to ignore to its detriment. Traditional Western medicine has its value and place. I am simply sharing our experiences, what worked for us and what has not.

Before you make the same decision for yourself or your children, however, I feel obliged to point out that my experiences go against the conventional wisdom of mainstream medicine. You need to satisfy yourself that you are making the right decision if you forego conventional medical treatment, childhood vaccinations, and the other resources of mainstream medicine. Your own—and the life and health of your children—will depend on making the right choices, and no one can guarantee that you will experience the same good results that I did.

I strongly recommend that you consult conventional medical doctors before you make the decision to use these approaches so you will understand the risks of doing so.

Although I have made every effort to ensure the accuracy and completeness of the information in this book, neither I nor the publisher assume responsibility for errors, inaccuracies, omissions, or inconsistencies in this book, nor do we assume responsibility if you choose to use the same approaches that I used but do not achieve the same successful results.

I refer to various brand-name herbal remedies and my experience in using them. The brands and their manufacturers are mentioned for informational purposes only, and my book is not sponsored by or affiliated with any of these companies. All value judgments are my own opinion only.

I have omitted the names of the various medical practitioners whom I consulted in seeking treatment for my son. All of my comments on people, places, products, or organizations are statements of my own opinion only.

A percentage of the profits after taxes from the sale of this book will be donated to charity, including but not limited to autism and vaccine damage awareness charities.

What Was It Like to Write This Book?

It was a calling, a mission, an assignment.

I kept thinking when Clay was sick, "I need to be writing this down." But I was too tired and too stressed. When I had the time and energy to work, it needed to go toward my real job.

After he recovered, I knew I needed to write our story, because it's not just our story. It's the story of a million other children and their families, and their struggle to survive.

It was great and painful.

The first draft practically wrote itself. The words just poured out of me. I would sit down at the computer, and it felt like the next time I looked up, hours had passed.

Then I got Clay's medical records from the pediatrician. Reading them was very painful. As I lived our relationship with the pediatrician I was frustrated. I knew Clay was very sick—it wasn't just back-to-back colds—but the pediatrician didn't believe me. I was looking to her as an expert on children's health. I expected her to be able to help Clay, and she never did. As I read the medical records, I relived all those horrible experiences.

Then I became angry. How could she be so blind? How could she put my son at risk like that, when everything was pointing to autism? Why didn't she know more about the subject? How could she give my son shots that were incubated in eggs when he was extremely allergic to eggs? I remember reading about autism on the American Academy of Pediatrics website, which said, if the parent thinks there is something wrong, there probably is. Nevertheless, she didn't believe me. Thank you, God, for leading me away from her and to someone who could help. I have done a lot of forgiveness work on the subject; I had to forgive myself, the pediatricians, and the pharmaceutical companies. I continue to forgive in this matter.

I have written other books: on table manners, football, and golf. They all seem pretty fluffy in comparison. Editing was more difficult with this book because I had to read the pages over and over again to make sure every word was perfect. With every word, I relived those two long years of Clay's illness. There are parts that make me cry every time I read them.

Writing this book also made me grateful. Clay has been healthy for a long time now; I sometimes take it for granted. Committing this story to paper vividly reminded me of how bad things really were, how miserable we all were, and how desperate I was to find answers. I always want to be grateful for this miraculous gift.

I have also found I am attracting people into my life who have the same problems we had. If you're reading this, you or someone you love probably has aluminum, yeast, parasites, or reverse polarity. Every person I meet who shares one of those issues teaches me something. I was working on a friend who kept testing positive for aluminum. I would release it, then go back and test another day, and the aluminum would still be there. I thought there was something wrong with what I was doing. Then she told me she was taking a prescription drug for her thyroid called Synthroid. I was told it was loaded with aluminum, so I looked it up in the *Physician's Desk Reference (PDR).* It listed 20 different aluminum ingredients. No wonder I couldn't clear her aluminum: She was putting it back into her body every day. She switched to Armour Thyroid, which according to the *PDR* is aluminum-free.

It seems that everyone I meet is sick or has a sick family member. Crohn's, cancer, lupus, and Alzheimer's are all curable, yet many do not want to do what is necessary to heal and recover. It is so frustrating. Many of those diseases are curable without the dangerous side effects of pharmaceuticals; however, so few are willing to try. Then there are the sick children I meet and hear about. I can see so many of them going down the same road Clay traveled. Their parents continue to give them the shots, every time risking a permanent regression into autism. I have had to learn to wait for the pregnant moment when a person is really open to hearing me. Many people I meet don't want help. Even though they or someone they love is ill, they stay with mainstream medicine, overlooking the fact it's not working and is actually making them sicker. It breaks my heart. I want a t-shirt that says, "*Please* don't tell me about your health problems if you're not willing to do something about them."

Then, of course, there is autism, the condition that touches my heart the most. It strikes our children, and they can't protect themselves. We can make great progress to reduce their symptoms and behaviors, but unfortunately a cure for autism still eludes us.

One unforeseen benefit to writing this book was it gave me a voice. While Clay was sick, I would talk to people about it. They would say, "That's normal; all kids bang their heads." Well, it wasn't natural. I never felt like people were really hearing me or appreciating how much trouble we were having—not even my closest friends and family.

I remember telling a friend the doctor had said Clay was at risk for autism. She didn't even bat an eye. She just went on talking about something else. I thought to myself, "Did you not hear me? My son might be autistic! Do you have any idea what that means?" But of course, she did not.

Many people thought I was neurotic about what Clay could eat and drink. They just didn't comprehend the consequences to his physical and emotional health. I am still told I'm too picky, but I'm not willing to go down that path again just so he can have a diet soda in a can.

Now that I've written this story and some of my loved ones have read it, they really understand how hard things were. Several people have said, "I'm so sorry. I knew Clay was sick, I just didn't know how bad it was. I wish I would have been there more." It feels good to know this has touched them.

It was still hard to share so much personal information with the world, to make our lives and our struggles—and my bad decisions—so public. I have a lot of regrets, and there are things I've written that embarrass me, but if they felt important to the story, I included them.

I have worried about how Clay is going to feel about this when he's old enough to read and understand this. Will it hurt his feelings? Will he feel guilty when he reads how difficult those years were for us? Will he be angry at me for letting them give him those shots? I have said a lot of prayers this book will bless him and complete his healing journey.

It's also frightening to write about something so unconventional. Many people accept stories of healing in the Bible; nevertheless, most do not believe it can happen today. Healing *does* take place today. God still works miracles. I know, because I've lived them. And they do remind me of the Bible, because there weren't any theatrics; it was all quiet and simple.

Religious Differences

I talk about God and Jesus in this book. If you are of another faith, please feel free to use the name of your divinity instead. The story of our illness and recovery is too important to be overlooked because of religious differences.

For the Skeptics

Our journey was a painful one. We explored every avenue we could find, starting with traditional Western medicine. As each treatment failed to produce results, we sought out others. I became extremely open-minded and would have done almost anything that was moral to find a cure for my son.

You, the reader, may not have traveled down as many rabbit holes as I have. It may be more difficult for you to embrace the healing art that was our final savior. If you need help, what harm can it do to suspend your disbelief or scepticism and try it? No matter what your faith, or lack thereof, it has worked for me and many others.

Science isn't always the answer. Science has an important role in the world, but this type of healing works with the mystery, power, and beauty of nature of which we are a part and which our technologically oriented society tends to ignore to its detriment.

Traditional Western medicine also has its value and place. I am simply sharing our experiences in this book, what worked for us and what has not.

1 "He's Not Autistic, But..."

- For no apparent reason, he bangs his head on window ledges, asphalt, the floor, and with his hands.

- He frequently walks on his toes, and sometimes spins in circles.

- He's extremely allergic to milk, corn, soy, eggs, oats, chocolate, feathers, and dust. Those are just the things we know he's allergic to. Eating is like walking through a minefield; we never know when something is going to cause an allergic reaction. Luckily he's not allergic to wheat, although people keep trying to get us to take him off of it because so many autistic children are allergic to wheat. Someone said to me, "I'm glad he just has allergies." But those allergies ruled our lives and destroyed his immune system and emotional state.

- He's two years old and can only say about eight things, mostly, *no, bu* for ball (which he uses to describe almost everything), and *du* for dad. A two-year-old should have a 50-word vocabulary and be using two-word sentences. At nine months old he used to say *mama* or randomly string noises together to make words, but that skill is long gone.

- He's sick most of the time and a cold means at least two weeks of hell for the whole family.

- His nose and chest are constantly congested, and mucous shoots down to his chest when he sneezes.

- He doesn't sleep for more than two or three hours at a time, waking frequently and crying.

- He's unhappy most of the time, grunting and crying; smiling is rare.

- He wants to be held all the time and refuses to walk even though he's capable; Mommy's back hurts most of the time as a result.

- He insists on climbing up on the bar in the den every night, and paces back and forth endlessly. It doesn't actually make him happy; he's just less unhappy. He grunts as he does it. Every night feels like a test of endurance.

- He absolutely hates to ride in the car. A fifteen-minute drive puts Mommy in a full sweat, and an hour drive is almost out of the question.

- We have to cut his hair when he sleeps because he becomes so hysterical and thrashes so much at the barber we're afraid he'll get hurt.

- Noises frighten him so much we carry a headset intended for a gun range in our diaper bag. Live performances, such as Barney, are out of the question because we can't even get him in the auditorium, much less sit through a performance. His hearing is so sensitive, he can hear one of us pull in the driveway before our dog does. The dog barking can set him off. A lawn mower backfiring during one of our walks can start a complete meltdown that will ruin the rest of the day for him. Many people think this is some type of gift we should embrace. People think it's cool because they've never had to live with it. One doctor said, "Maybe he can be one of those guys who sits on submarines and listens for bombs." We don't want our son to suffer from these bizarre sensory integration issues.

- The tags in his clothes bother him to the point we have to surgically remove them from every shirt to make sure no plastic thread or part of the tag is left to rub his skin. He won't wear shirts with snaps, even though they're easier to get on over his head, because something about the snaps bothers him.

- His shoelaces have to be tied backwards, because he wants them exactly perpendicular to his leg. He becomes explosive if I forget and hurriedly tie them my normal way.

- He has systemic yeast.

- He makes eye contact, although I frequently find him looking through me instead of at me.

- He likes to watch fans, although not as much as he did when he was a baby.

- He sometimes crawls on the floor on his hands and knees and bizarrely drags his head as he moves across the floor.

2 The Doctor Says He's at Risk for Autism

"He's not autistic, but…" I kept hearing myself say as I explained Clay's behavior, illnesses, inability to sleep through the night, and sensory issues. I hated the way it sounded; it automatically made everyone think he *was* autistic. But the similarities he shared with the autistic spectrum explained so much about his behavior.

His doctor said, "A child like Clay who is at risk for autism shouldn't have vaccines."

I felt like he had hit me in the stomach with a baseball bat. I had feared autism since he started banging his head at age one. To hear the word autism come out of a doctor's mouth when I hadn't brought it up was terrifying. I responded, "My husband is going to ask me why he's at risk for autism.…"

"Well, I wouldn't label him like that, but he does share a biomedical spectrum of disorders with the autistic," he responded. It was too late; he had already told me my son was *at risk for autism*. I was scared stiff.

This was a new doctor for Clay, a specialist in lost causes: chronic fatigue, fibromyalgia, autism, cancer, and immune disorders. I even met someone in his office who had the Ebola virus. He was the first M.D. to admit there was something wrong with Clay. I told him about trying to work with Clay's pediatrician and how she kept telling me he was fine. He responded, "He's not fine, he's far from fine." Although it was validating to finally have a doctor admit something was wrong, it was also terrifying.

His new doctor said Clay was not producing growth hormone, and he wasn't absorbing the nutrients from the food he ate. He put him on melatonin for sleep, a liquid multivitamin that is very popular for autistic children, probiotics, nystatin, and Diflucan for the yeast.

He wanted to do more tests, but I refused. Clay was already completely freaked out by doctors' offices, and he has a memory like a steel trap. When the doctor met him for the first time and saw how hysterical Clay became just being in a doctor's office, he agreed Clay did not need to come in again unless something unusual required his physical presence.

3 *Allergens*

Most autistic children have food allergies—typically milk, corn, soy, eggs, and wheat, the big five allergens. People kept trying to get me to take him off wheat and do the gluten-free/casein-free diet, which is so popular for autistic children, But I had done my homework on allergies, and I knew Clay wasn't allergic to wheat. I wasn't about to restrict his diet any more than it already was.

At age two, Clay's allergies were the focus of my attention because he was severely allergic. His symptoms would come on quickly and sometimes violently. If he ate eggs, he would projectile vomit; if he got batter with eggs in it on his skin, he would break out in a rash. Anything with cow's milk in it would cause profuse and immediate mucous; he couldn't even eat cheese. Table salt coming in contact with his skin would cause hives, and chocolate would cause immediate head-banging and toe-walking. Oats would cause his face to flush and his ears to get red. Feathers and dust caused sneezing and tons of mucous.

Because I was breastfeeding, I also had to give up most of these allergens. If I were to slip up, the consequences were quite painful. One night at a wedding, I had ice cream with the wedding cake. Ice cream has milk in it, but because I so rarely eat it, it didn't dawn on me. Clay nursed when I got home, woke up in the middle of the night, and was up half the night crying and restless because of his allergic reaction to the cow's milk in my breast milk.

The more strictly I kept him on an allergy-free diet, the less likely he was to head-bang and toe-walk. It also reduced but did not eliminate the mucous. The head-banging was always one of the final symptoms, indicating to me his system was on overload. His body was telling me, "I'm miserable; I can't take any more, make this pain go away." Most of the pictures from when he was one year old show bruises on his forehead because that was when he started banging his head, and before I discovered all of his allergies. Those pictures still make me sad.

When we would vacation with my family, and Clay would continually be exposed to small amounts of allergens, he would be banging his head and walking on his toes by the end of the week. His sleep would be even more disturbed than normal, and he would be grumpier than usual. It would take days for him to settle down after our return.

I carried tissues with me all the time because his snot would shoot down to his chest when he sneezed. My robes were always covered in mucous, because he was the worst in the morning.

Every morning I would lay in bed with my hand on his chest, feeling and listening to his labored breathing and the gurgling mucous in his chest and nose and pray for a miracle. I knew I would do what was necessary to get him healthy, if I could just find out what that was. I kept feeling like there was someone—or something—out there who was going to be able to help. That's why I kept looking.

4 Yeast

Clay had systemic yeast, another typical problem for autistic children. But the test did show a healthy amount of acidophilus in his digestive tract, which the doctor was very surprised about. I presume this was because we had been giving Clay powdered acidophilus with at least one meal a day for about a year, and he loved it. We would put it on his nut butter sandwiches. Because it was sweet, he would actually eat it with a spoon. Acidophilus is the friendly bacteria found in our digestive tract. Normally an absence of acidophilus is associated with a yeast overgrowth. Acidophilus is also referred to as a probiotic.

There are whole books written about yeast overgrowths, and there is a great deal of discussion about it in the alternative health and autistic community. Healthy people have a balance of both yeast and good bacteria in their digestive system. The predominant thinking is when a person takes antibiotics, they kill the good bacteria in the digestive tract along with the bad bacteria they are intended to kill. This makes the digestive tract susceptible to a yeast overgrowth. The good bacteria are called beneficial bacteria, and they help with the digestive process.

When the yeast grows out of control because of a lack of beneficial bacteria, bad things happen. The yeast can spread from the digestive system to the rest of the body, causing a systemic yeast infection. The yeast becomes a parasite rather than a balancing friend.

Yeast needs sugar to grow and survive; it then creates alcohol as a waste product. My brother-in-law describes it not so eloquently as, "Yeast eats sugar and poops alcohol." That's why it's used in the production of beer and wine. As a result, a person with a yeast overgrowth will crave refined carbohydrates, and then be tired after eating them because of the alcohol waste caused by the yeast organisms. This too causes extreme mood swings because of the imbalances it causes in the bloodstream.

Yeast causes many symptoms; some are similar to the symptoms of parasites, because the yeast becomes parasitic. A simple way to describe it is a person with a yeast overgrowth is uncomfortable in his own skin. They itch, they're moody, they have intense cravings, their energy level can vary dramatically, and they don't sleep well. A person suffering from a yeast overgrowth is living on a roller coaster—one caused by the metabolic process of the yeast organism's need to eat and create waste.

There are many diets, prescriptions, herbs, homeopathic remedies, and probiotics that are recommended for a yeast overgrowth. You can go on a strict yeast diet, and take all the products you can find, but you won't get rid of the underlying cause of the yeast until you get rid of the aluminum. If you have a yeast overgrowth, you have aluminum. Yeast *always* means aluminum is or was present. It doesn't always go the other way, however, as it is possible to have aluminum without having a yeast overgrowth.

Aluminum kills bacteria. That's why it's used so widely as a preservative. When you have aluminum in your system, it kills the beneficial bacteria, allowing a yeast overgrowth. Antibiotics are loaded with aluminum, plus they kill the beneficial bacteria in your digestive system. Antibiotics are wonderful for serious infections but absolutely must be used wisely, and of course they should never be taken for a virus, because they have no effect on a virus. If you take antibiotics for an extended period, like many people do for acne, you will undoubtedly end up with both aluminum and yeast.

Aluminum was the underlying problem for both Clay and me. It causes many problems, and I have yet to find a book or website that makes it clear how dangerous aluminum is or adequately describes the many problems it sets in motion, such as yeast. (I will discuss aluminum in greater detail in its own section.)

If you have a yeast overgrowth, you have to get rid of the aluminum first. Then you can go on a yeast diet and finally get the overgrowth under control.

5 His Frequent Illnesses

Clay was ill most of the time. If he came anywhere near someone with a respiratory infection, Clay would get it, and the next two weeks would be horrible. After those two weeks, it would only be tolerable, not gone. His colds seemed to last forever.

Sometimes he would get so sick he would just sit in my lap and whimper all day. He was miserable. We ended up at the emergency room on a couple of Saturdays because he wouldn't stop crying, and something was obviously very wrong. They did X-rays, a catheter, took blood, and made a sick baby even more miserable than he already was. On one occasion, they believed he was constipated, so they sent us home with enemas, even though his bowels were moving every day.

I was afraid all the attention he was getting was causing him to be sick. I prayed I wasn't causing his illness, and that he wasn't either. I worried about the Florence Nightingale effect, where the caretaker causes the illness in order to feel needed. In addition, I was concerned about Clay becoming dependent on me because I was always there when he was ill.

My husband would get mad at me because I would send the nanny home when Clay was sick. "You need a break!" he would say heatedly. I just couldn't leave him with someone else when he was really sick and needed me. He would scream and cry anytime he was taken from me. Sometimes in the morning my husband would take him downstairs so I could get another hour of sleep. Clay would cry hysterically when he was taken from me, then sit at the bottom of the steps and cry until I came down. It was awful.

Clay was very dependent on me, and I was getting little sleep. I felt like I did nothing but take care of an ill child, sleep, and work. When he was willing to let my husband take care of him, the only thing I wanted to do was sleep.

6 Where Did It All Start?

What made Clay so sick? He seemed fine when we came home from the hospital, and he slept well, although his sensitivity to sound was already there. If we opened a soda can in the same room with him, he would wake up crying. We didn't know the canned diet soda I was drinking at the time was contributing to both his illness and mine. At this point in time, we didn't even know I was sick, although there were plenty of signs.

By the time he was three weeks old, he was no longer sleeping well, and he was unhappy most of the time.

We were later to find out his illness started with me. I was the carrier for his underlying problem, which turned out to be aluminum. I passed it on to him while he was in the womb and while I was breastfeeding. We furthermore continued to contaminate him and me with aluminum in a number of ways after he was born:

- Consuming things packaged in aluminum cans and foil
- Taking prescription and nonprescription medication that contained aluminum
- Cooking with aluminum cookware
- Getting a flu shot every year, which contains aluminum and other toxins
- Baby shots, or vaccines, which contain aluminum
- Using toothpaste packaged in aluminum
- Consuming table salt and baking soda, which are two of a number of other ways aluminum gets into our bodies

The prescriptions for antihistamines, steroids, antibiotics, and decongestants the pediatrician gave him made him even sicker, because most of them contain aluminum. This, along with the other ingredients, such as the stimulants in the decongestants, were more than his toxic little body could handle. Unfortunately, I didn't know all this at the time because I wouldn't knowingly give my son something that would hurt him.

He had parasites as well, which by themselves create havoc, but in combination with aluminum made him miserable. These didn't surface until after the aluminum was cleared. The body can only heal so much at one time. If you try to do too much, you can bring on a healing crisis, where a new illness, disease, or symptom is brought on by giving the body more work than it can handle. Some people in the alternative community think this is a normal part of healing. I prefer to avoid a healing crisis, and instead work at a pace my body can comfortably tolerate.

I have seen other children diagnosed with both aluminum and parasites at the same time, but they were not as sick as Clay was from the aluminum. Releasing Clay's aluminum was a huge change and improvement for him; then clearing the parasites brought him the rest of the way back to good health.

7 Mommy's Infertility and Preeclampsia

I didn't know I was sick until long after my son became sick. Although looking back on it, there were plenty of signs I didn't understand.

My fertility problems first became apparent when I was 35, which pointed to an underlying health problem. Unfortunately, the doctors I saw said it was simply premature ovarian failure, with no known cause and no cure or treatment available. I would later find out aluminum, which made both my son and me so sick, causes infertility as well. It settles in the solar plexus and causes the organs, including the uterus, to drop. As a result, it can be almost impossible to become pregnant.

I became pregnant for the first time at age 39 after years of trying to have a child. I tried all the fertility treatments, including temperature charts, hormone pills, hormone shots, and in vitro fertilization. I was thrilled to finally be pregnant and enjoyed the doctor visits to learn how the baby was doing.

I had frequent and intense headaches by the time I was two months pregnant and began having a great deal of swelling in my ankles at three months. I spent most evenings on the couch with my feet propped up trying to get the swelling to go down. By the time I was five months pregnant, my ankles were swollen all the time and looked like tree trunks.

At week 28, I had a dizzy spell, and my blood pressure was elevated. After a 24-hour test that measures protein in the urine, I was diagnosed with toxemia, or preeclampsia. Preeclampsia is a condition in pregnancy characterized by abrupt hypertension (a sharp rise in blood pressure); leakage of large amounts of protein into the urine; and edema (swelling) of the hands, feet, and face. I was restricted to bed rest. My obstetrician told me "the exact causes of toxemia are not known."

I was terrified because the only woman I had ever personally known with toxemia died from it. I remember going to her funeral. Her face and neck were so swollen I would not have recognized her. In her situation, the illness escalated after the child was born, which is rare. Normally the condition stabilizes as soon as the baby is born. I was soon to find out my mother had toxemia too, and in her case, the baby died.

Every time my blood pressure would spiral up, I would fear the worst for me and my baby. I called my attorney to see if I could get a will put together quickly in case I didn't make it. My illness made the rest of my pregnancy very emotional and intimidating.

In the world of alternative healthcare there are treatments available for toxemia, but I didn't know that at the time. Some alternative doctors believe toxemia is simply a magnesium imbalance, which can be monitored and prevented. When it spirals out of control, hospitals will give you magnesium IVs. The goal is to prevent it from getting that far. When I told my obstetrician this during my second pregnancy, she agreed toxemia is a magnesium imbalance. So why on earth didn't she put me on magnesium during my last pregnancy, when I had toxemia?

During my second pregnancy, three years after Clay's birth, I took magnesium whenever I experienced swelling, and I took quite a bit of it on and off as needed.

I also experienced the worst constipation of my life following my son's birth. I now know a magnesium deficiency causes constipation, hence Milk of Magnesia. When I have any signs of constipation, I take magnesium, and it quickly remedies the problem.

Some herbalists believe toxemia is caused by a malfunction in the spleen, where the uric acid is out of balance and cannot be released. Safflowers are the remedy used to prevent or cure toxemia in this case.

The symptoms of toxemia are the kidneys stop functioning properly, causing high blood pressure, violent headaches, protein in the urine, and excessive swelling in the feet, ankles, hands, neck, and face. The condition can escalate to the point where it causes permanent damage to the eyes, kidneys, and liver. The final stages of the disease can cause seizures and can be fatal for both the mother and the baby.

I originally responded very well to bed rest, losing several pounds of water weight over the weekend. My blood pressure dropped, and the swelling disappeared. Over the next two months, however, my blood pressure yo-yoed up and down and the swelling came back.

I was given steroid injections to assist in the baby's lung development. The doctor did an amniocentesis to check the progress. At week 37, my doctor convinced me to induce labor, which was unsuccessful. She broke my water, taking the pregnancy to the point of no return, and I ended up having a cesarean-section.

P-gel and Pitocin were both used to induce labor. I later found out how dangerous Pitocin is to the unborn baby. It causes the baby to thrust against the labor canal and pelvic bones much more forcefully and rapidly than would occur under normal birthing conditions. The baby's head is soft and not protected from this unnatural force. Pitocin has been linked to autism and other learning disorders. For instance, my osteopath's daughter has permanent brain damage to the right occipital lobe and a permanent learning disability, caused by Pitocin and the artificial thrust it created during birth. As a result, during my last pregnancy, I did not allow them to induce labor. The risk is too great.

I later discovered that women who have toxemia, induced labor, or a C-section are all at higher risk for having a child with autism than the general population. Of course, no one told me that. I didn't find out until after my son had recovered.

I actually became the most ill following the birth, which as I mentioned, is rare. My blood pressure reached 185/110 (normal is 120/80). I was told by the doctor I was at risk for a stroke. I thought to myself, "I can't have a stroke; I have a baby to take care of!" There were times in my life when I would have felt like my death would be no great loss. This was not one of those times.

The headaches were awful and the swelling ridiculous. I looked like I had elephant legs. They were worse than at any time during my pregnancy, which I wouldn't have thought possible. Bed rest would have helped, and so would have magnesium or safflowers, but I didn't know that at the time. I was put on high blood pressure medication to control my symptoms.

Four weeks later, the swelling was gone, and my blood pressure was normal; nevertheless, I was kept on the high blood pressure meds for a year.

Shortly after the birth of my son, I had a complete workup by a cardiologist. He found no underlying problems with my heart or circulatory system, or cause for my high blood pressure. The whole thing was puzzling because I had previously had low blood pressure. By the time I was finally taken off the medicine, I was having dizzy spells from low blood pressure.

Clay's Health at Birth

While I was pregnant, I had numerous ultrasounds and an amniocentesis because of my advanced maternal age and toxemia. Clay hiccupped a lot while in the womb. I now know the frequent hiccupping indicated he was allergic to things I was eating and drinking. He continued to hiccup frequently after he came home from the hospital.

He was given a vaccine in the hospital when he was one day old, and he had the usual baby shots at four weeks old, with four in one day.

8 *Nursing*

This section is a rather graphic description of our breastfeeding problems. If it will bother you, feel free to skip to the next section.

I was nursing, which was quite a challenge. Nursing should not hurt. I had trouble nursing and had pain because I was sick and had aluminum, which leads to a yeast overgrowth. Yeast makes nursing agonizing. Unfortunately, you can't completely clear up the yeast until you get rid of the aluminum. The yeast is always lurking under the surface when you have aluminum.

Every time my son latched on, it felt like my nipple was being slammed in a car door. It made me gasp for breath. My husband thought it was funny, although I certainly didn't. Eventually, during each nursing session, the hurting would lessen, but it still hurt throughout and would reintensify when he switched breasts. I saw a lactation consultant and went to La Leche meetings, but no one could help. (La Leche is a support group for nursing mothers. It offers an immense depth of knowledge on the subject.) His latch was fine, but I was still in agony.

I used a nipple shield, even though all the nursing books say you shouldn't. For me it was a question of using a shield or the fear I wouldn't stick it out, and might end up resorting to formula. I had several shields and kept one hidden in my bra. I was deathly afraid he would want to nurse and I wouldn't have one. The pain without the shield was almost unbearable.

By three weeks old he was nursing nonstop from 8 P.M. until midnight. This would later extend from 6 P.M. until midnight, and became a nightly ritual for several months.

He became quite colicky following his four-week shots. Neverthe-less, I didn't put two and two together and see the relationship to the shots. By the time he was six weeks old, he would cry from 5:00 P.M. until midnight. The only thing that made him somewhat happy was to nurse, so we would frequently nurse from 6:00 P.M. until midnight. I couldn't even get up to go to the bathroom without him shrieking the whole two minutes I was gone. I remember nursing him on the kitchen counter so I could eat my dinner.

His foul humor continued for the next two years.

Unfortunately, we gave him the standard vaccines until he was about 15 months old. Luckily, we never gave him the MMR, which stands for measles, mumps, and rubella, and I thank God almost every day for sparing us.

Breastfeeding finally became comfortable at about eight weeks, and I abandoned the shield. It was such a relief; I felt like a real breastfeeding mom. In breastfeeding circles, there is a sense of shame using a nipple shield, and I was happy to be free of it.

Clay refused solid food until he was a year old and continued to nurse intensely the whole time. Refusal to eat solid food is considered a sign of sensory integration issues, which would certainly surface later. These issues are associated with the autistic spectrum.

When Clay was a little over one year old, I was pumping my breast milk at work, and there was a burning in my breast ducts. I instinctively knew it was a yeast infection because I had experienced vaginal yeast infections, and the burning was familiar. The following day when I pumped, there was blood in my milk. There was nothing obvious, such as antibiotics, that precipitated this yeast infection. It just seemed to come out of nowhere.

I called my La Leche League leader and discussed the subject. She was a huge help and confirmed that, yes, you can have a yeast infection in your breast ducts. She suggested a prescription antifungal I was able to get from my doctor, although my doctor would only give me two doses, and I eventually discovered I needed much more.

My La Leche leader suggested gentian violet, which can be pur-chased over the counter but frequently has to be ordered. It was horribly messy and stained both my breasts and my son's face. It turned my pumped milk a disgusting shade of light purple. The combination of the prescription antifungal and gentian violet seemed to cure the yeast infection almost immediately.

Six months later I had to take antibiotics for an infection, and the yeast infection started all over again, but this time it was much worse. The pain during nursing was intense. Every time he would latch on I could hardly breathe, like someone was smashing my nipple with a hammer. It felt just like it did when he was born. It made me wonder if the pain I had for the first eight weeks had been an undiagnosed yeast infection.

I developed an open sore on my nipple, which Clay made worse every time he latched on. I tried the nipple shield, but by now, he would have nothing to do with it. I had to put a bandage on my nipple, which he hated, but I couldn't survive without it. There was blood in my breast milk again and pumping was torture. I tried the gentian violet again, but this time the problem was too big.

By now I was seeing a doctor who was much more versed on the difficulty of clearing up a systemic yeast overgrowth. I was predisposed to yeast problems because I took antibiotics to treat acne for several years while I was in high school. As I would later find out, I had aluminum, which is always present when there is a yeast overgrowth. Aluminum sets you up to be constantly at risk for yeast problems because of its antibiotic properties.

A simple blood test confirmed I had significantly elevated antibodies to *Candida* (the scientific name for one type of yeast), indicating I had systemic yeast. Systemic yeast is simply a yeast overgrowth throughout the body. Based on my test results, medical history, and symptoms, my doctor believed I had been experiencing a yeast overgrowth for a very long time.

I spent five months taking Diflucan, nystatin, and probiotics before the blood tests confirmed the yeast overgrowth was under control. Diflucan is a powerful antifungal, which helps with systemic yeast. Nystatin is an antifungal that works solely in the digestive tract where a yeast overgrowth normally starts. I had taken Diflucan with my previous yeast infection, but my old doctor was only willing to give me two pills. This time I ended up taking one a day for five months, which is quite expensive at about ten dollars a pill. Probiotics, such as acidophilus, are the beneficial bacteria that live in our digestive tract. By taking them, I was reintroducing the beneficial bacteria back into my system.

I went on a very strict yeast diet, which pretty much reduced what I could eat to meat, nuts, and vegetables for 30 days. What we eat and drink contributes to yeast because it requires sugar and refined carbohydrates to survive.

The same doctor put my son on antifungals and probiotics so we wouldn't be passing the yeast infection back and forth.

9 Chronology of Clay's Pediatrician Visits

This chapter is a time line of Clay's pediatrician visits and my calls on his behalf. It jumps ahead of the rest of the story, where we will later come back and fill in some of the blanks as to what was happening outside of the pediatrician's office. As I was reading his medical records, there was a clear pattern that only comes out if you look at our interaction with the doctor instance after instance. The pattern I saw was I was concerned about his upper respiratory problems, allergies, and immune disorders, and the pediatrician was worried about giving him his next shot. Clay frequently became more ill shortly after each shot. I asked repeatedly about his constant illnesses, and she continually blew off my concerns and said he was normal, which he was not.

The pediatrician came to our hospital room when Clay was one day old and gave him the first hepatitis B shot. He had mild facial jaundice.

At two weeks old, I asked our pediatrician about the link between the MMR (the combination shot for measles, mumps, and rubella) and autism. My cousin in Ireland, who is a nurse, had told me about the link. She didn't give her children any of the shots. Our pediatrician became angry and adamantly defended all the baby shots. She was not open to discussion on the subject, and unfortunately, I believed her because of her emotional conviction.

At our four-week pediatric visit, she and I discussed my concerns about his congestion and disrupted sleep. Although he was sick, they still gave him the second hepatitis B shot.

At two months old, despite his still-active cough, he was given four more shots, one of which (the DTaP) was a combination, meaning it carries more than one virus: DTaP, IPV, HIB, and Prevnar. Two days later we needed Tylenol instructions faxed to the daycare center, and one week later we needed Pediacare for a cold. He was fussy but no fever.

When Clay was three months old, I called about a flu shot, in hopes it would prevent these respiratory illnesses. I was told I could have one, which I got, with the intention of protecting Clay, but Clay had to wait until he was six months old. My allergist had convinced me years earlier I had to get a flu shot every year because of my predisposition to bronchitis and laryngitis. He believed in addition to preventing the flu, the shots prevented many upper-respiratory infections. When I did get my flu shot, I got fewer respiratory infections, so there seemed to be a relationship to me, which I hoped would help my son.

At three and a half months old we needed the Pediacare (for congestion) and Mylicon (for gas) instructions faxed to the daycare center again.

At four months old, Clay came down with croup. It was horrible. He ended up on antibiotics and steroids, and was sick most of the time for the next nineteen months.

Four days after he developed croup and was still very sick, they wanted to give him more shots. I refused them until he was healthier. In addition, they believed he had viral bronchitis.

At five months old he was given his four-month shots, DTaP #2, IPV #2, HIB #2, and Prevnar #2, even though he was still sick.

At his six-month visit I talked to the doctor about Clay's constant congestion and mucous. I asked if it could be allergies. She said, "No, it's an immune response. He can't develop allergies until he's one year old." He had been sick now for two solid months, yet his father and I were healthy. He hadn't been exposed to anyone who had been ill. The doctor said he'd been having back-to-back colds, which I found hard to believe. We had taken him out of daycare and were keeping him at home with us. Where was he getting these viruses? It's not as though he got well and then sick again; he had been constantly sick for two months. In spite of all this, they gave him four more shots: DTaP #3, HIB #3, Prevnar #3, and a flu shot. At this point in time, I was still a supporter of flu shots and had hoped this shot would make Clay more able to resist upper-respiratory infections. That was not to be the case.

One week after these last shots his illness took a turn for the worse. Over the weekend we ended up in the emergency room. They believed it was RSV, or respiratory syncytial virus, which in children can cause severe pulmonary diseases including bronchiolitis and pneumonia. He also had an ear infection, so they gave him antibiotics, a prescription cough syrup, and Proventil. He was irritable, had labored breathing, a hoarse cough—but no fever.

We saw the pediatrician the following Monday. She believed it was RSV even though the test was negative. She said the test had to be done in a precise manner, and they probably didn't do it correctly at the hospital. I had no desire to have it done again since he was in no mood to cooperate, so she treated it without another test. He wasn't sleeping and was wheezing. She changed his prescriptions and was upset about the ones he was given at the hospital. "First of all, do no harm," she said angrily about what they gave him and added a short dosage of antihistamines. I would later find her statement cruelly ironic since she was part of the medical community pushing the shots that contributed so greatly to his illness.

At seven months old, he got his second flu shot. By this time his ears seemed better.

A week after his second flu shot he had blood in his bowel movement, and less than two weeks later he was croupy again.

At nine months old, we started seeing another doctor in the pediatric group who was a supporter of breastfeeding, and I again asked about vaccine safety. She was much more open to at least *hearing* my concerns. She gave me a book, which I read, and we decided to simply limit future shots to one per week. She reassured me their vaccines were mercury-free, which I was later to find out was not true. Some of their vaccines did contain mercury.

At ten months old, Clay got the Hep #3. The appointment called for two shots; we refused one. The nurse was not happy with me because she had already drawn both. Two weeks later Clay got the IPV #3 shot. Two days after the IPV shot I called the doctor because Clay was up most of the night, had nasal congestion, and was pulling at his ears.

We saw the pediatrician just after Clay's first birthday and discussed the fact his nose was constantly runny. In spite of this, he was still given the varicella vaccine, but thank goodness not the MMR, which was called for at the time.

A week after the varicella shot we were back at the pediatrician's because Clay's symptoms were worse, including congestion, not sleeping, difficulty breathing through his nose, difficulty feeding, and sneezing. The doctor *finally* admitted Clay might have allergies and prescribed an antihistamine.

A few days later we called the pediatrician because he still wasn't sleeping, he was congested, and having trouble nursing. They changed antihistamines.

A week later we saw the pediatrician again because he still wasn't sleeping. Clay was also coughing, nasally, and snotty. They recommended nasal steroids, which we refused, and they changed the antihistamines again.

When Clay was 14 months old, we ended up at the ER on a Saturday morning because he was crying uncontrollably. He appeared to be having abdominal pain. He had a fever. We were told, "His chest X-ray is normal, heart size is normal, and lungs appear clear. Skeletal structures appear intact and there are no unusual calcifications." They of course asked us if he was current on his vaccines, which he wasn't because of the MMR, although I wasn't about to tell them.

They did a catheter to get a clean urine sample, an abdominal X-ray, and blood work. They decided he had mild constipation and sent us home with enemas. It was a very unpleasant experience for my son and for us. He was already a wreck, and the hours in the ER and the tests put him over the edge. Giving him the enemas was a nightmare.

We saw the pediatrician on Monday, following the ER visit, and she wanted to give him more vaccines, even though we still didn't know what was wrong with him, and he'd been lethargic and crying for going on three days now. I declined the shots because he was so sick. The nurse called me later after she received the records from the ER and told me he had a sizeable impaction of 5 centimeters, which is about 2 inches. Even though he was having bowel movements, he was constipated. He spent the whole day in my lap whimpering. He finally had one of those huge breast-fed-baby bowel movements that night, and returned to his normal self. I would later find out constipation is frequently a sign of food allergies. Constipation and abnormal bowel movements are very common among autistic children. Clay had a history of only having one bowel movement per week, and on one occasion went 16 days between bowel movements.

A few weeks later we called about his upper respiratory problems again. He was sneezing with a runny nose, and we wanted to know if he could take something for the congestion.

When Clay was 15 months old, we called again about his upper-respiratory problems. This time it was nasal congestion, yellow mucous, runny nose, and a new cough. They offered us a flu shot, and we asked if he should get one while he's sick. We ended up waiting two weeks before he was given one. I asked the nurse about his head-banging, and she told me it was the start of the terrible twos. I did not agree. I was concerned the antihistamines might be causing it.

A few days later I saw the pediatrician in person and discussed my concerns about his head-banging. She suggested I take him off the anti-histamines if that's what I thought might be causing it. He had hardly slept at all for two days. She put him on antibiotics for his upper respi-ratory infection.

At 15 and a half months old, he was given a flu shot.

At about 16 months, he was given the DTaP, and the HIB #4. I don't know why I allowed him to have two shots on the same day, al-though that's what his medical records say. I talked to the doctor about his allergies too. I had determined by this time he was very allergic to cow's milk and all dairy products.

The day after these shots, he came down with thrush, and I devel-oped an awful yeast infection in my breasts. He was given nystatin, an antifungal.

At a year and a half, we were in Colorado, and he had a bad cold, so we gave him an over-the-counter cold remedy. He had a bad reaction to it, including difficulty breathing and a racing heart. We took him to the ER in the middle of the night. They were more concerned about his elevated heart rate than anything else.

When we got back home, we saw the pediatrician and told her about the incident in Colorado. I explained that by now I had discovered how extensive his allergies were:

- He's allergic to cow's milk, corn, soy, and eggs.
- He gets hives from topical contact with salt.
- He bangs his head after eating chocolate or being exposed to allergens.
- He toe-walks when he eats allergens.

Despite all of this, she was more concerned about his weight than his allergies or reaction to the cold medication. She suggested high-calorie foods, including cow's milk. When I reminded her he can't drink milk because he's allergic to it, she asked, "What happens when he drinks milk?" I felt like I had been talking to a brick wall. I had done all this research on allergies on my own. She had offered me no help on the subject. She didn't even suggest an elimination diet, much less allergy management of our environment. She didn't appear to understand the basics of allergies beyond prescribing an antihistamine. Now she was suggesting I feed him something he's allergic to so he could put on a half pound. He was in the fiftieth percentile for his age and weight, and I didn't agree with her his weight was a priority. It was the least of my concerns at the time.

She brought up the MMR on this visit, and I again declined. (Later on in this book I will explain how divine intervention the night before this doctor's visit made it clear to me he was never to have the MMR.)

My son had been almost constantly sick for over a year; he had frequent and sometimes fierce allergic reactions, but all she cared about was his weight and when he was going to get the MMR. I had talked to her about his upper-respiratory and immune problems on 22 separate occasions. She was ignoring the elephant crushing his chest. All she could do was nitpick her checklist of items, such as height and weight, and push her shots at the expense of my son's health.

It became apparent to me one of the advantages to the pediatric business is the children come in on a regular basis to get the scheduled shots. So the doctor is getting all of these office visits that would not normally occur with a healthy child. Additionally, there is the profit in the actual shots. It made her blind to the risks involved and to other serious issues, such as the immune problems my son had. All she could do was cookie-cutter doctoring that included shots, and height and weight measurements. I desperately needed help, and I wasn't getting it from her.

We went back a month later, and she was satisfied with his weight gain, but he was still very mucousy, flushed, and cranky. Of course, she thought it was normal and wasn't the least bit concerned about it.

I never took my son back to that pediatric group again.

10 Riding in the Car and Sensory Integration Issues

Clay absolutely hated riding in the car. When he was tiny and sleeping most of the time, riding in the car would often make him cry, which is unusual. Most children fall asleep when you put them in the car, but not Clay. It actually seemed to wake him up. We used to like to go out for breakfast—it was maybe a 15-minute drive—and I would sit in the backseat and nurse him the whole time so he wouldn't cry. Once we got there he would go to sleep.

Taking him anywhere at night was absolutely out of the question. I have no idea why things were so much worse at night, but they were—a hundred times worse. There was an evening La Leche League meeting about 15 minutes away from my house. I loved those meetings; it was a way for me to connect with other nursing mothers. It nourished my soul. The howling Clay did on the way, however, was not worth it.

The first time I went to a meeting, Clay cried and screamed the entire way there. I drove with my body twisted so I could shake a toy in front of him and keep one eye on the road. By the time I got there I was a wreck. As soon as we got out of the car, he was happy. The second time I asked my husband to drive us so I could sit in the back seat and entertain him. It didn't help at all. He still screamed and cried all the way there and back. Even taking him out of his car seat and holding him didn't help. He was still hysterical. The last time I attempted to go, I drove myself. I got about three minutes from the house, and he was in full-scale meltdown. I thought to myself, "What am I doing? This is torturing Clay. These meetings are supposed to bring Mommy and Baby together, but this drive is making us both absolutely miserable. Why am I doing this to us?" I turned around and went home, and never attempted to attend another evening meeting. Luckily there was a day-time meeting I ended up attending; unfortunately it was twice the distance.

At some point in time Clay decided he didn't like to have his diaper changed or his nose wiped. Later on I would discover these were sensory integration issues. When we even went near the area where he was to have his diaper changed, he would start screaming. Getting his diaper off and putting a clean one on him felt like varsity wrestling. Yes, I am bigger than he is; however, a hysterical baby has an amazing amount of strength, and I didn't want to hurt him. The bowel movement diapers were the worst. Breast-fed babies have huge, watery bowel movements, and with him thrashing all over the place it was practically impossible to keep his feet out of the mess.

Because he was constantly sick, his nose was always runny and caked with dried mucous. Wiping his nose was not okay with him. I hated seeing his nose like that, but it wasn't worth wiping it because it made him so mad, and it would just be a mess again within fifteen minutes. I remember trying to get the dried mucous out of his nostrils when he was asleep with tweezers, trying not to wake him up.

11 *Croup*

Clay developed croup when he was four months old. He had already been sick several times, but this was his first serious illness. This was when it became apparent to me something was wrong with his immune system. I took him out of daycare and kept him with me until he was old enough to have a flu shot, which I hoped would prevent his colds. It didn't work.

He was much more sickly than the other children at daycare. When they had a runny nose, he would get a cough and a fever, or in this case, croup. The other children seemed to fight off the viruses, but every single one he came in contact with brought him to his knees. His immune system was weaker than theirs; I just didn't know why.

Our pediatrician told us he was having back-to-back colds for six solid months following the croup. His nose was always filled with mucous, and his chest was gurgly too.

We finally ended up making the difficult decision to not take him out of the house until spring in an attempt to keep him healthy. We didn't take him out for the whole winter, not to the drugstore, not to dinner—I even went to La Leche League meetings by myself. I remember telling my La Leche group one day we were keeping Clay "quarantined" at home in an attempt to keep him healthy. Keeping him home was quite a burden; we felt trapped. Had it worked, it would have been worth it. But it didn't. Even though my husband and I were virus-free all winter, our son continued to be sick the entire time.

We decided to give him a flu shot at six months old in hopes it would help with his immune system. It did not. I remember thinking I needed to time the birth of our next baby to come at the beginning of spring so I didn't have to worry about cold and flu season.

I asked the doctor if it could be allergies because my husband and I both have a family tree filled with allergies and asthma. She said, "No, allergies are an immune response that doesn't develop until one year old." I now know this is not true: You can be born with allergies, as my son was.

12 *Vaccines*

Just prior to Clay's first birthday, a friend of my mom's, an acupuncturist, was visiting from out of town, and warned me about the vaccines. To me she sounded a little over the top, saying not to have any of the shots and criticizing the polio vaccine. I thought to myself, "Everybody knows the polio vaccine cured polio." I would later find out not everyone agrees with that statement. Many people believe polio had almost run its course. Similar to the plague, which eventually disappeared in Europe, polio was already on the decline when the vaccine was introduced.

She said to search on Amazon.com under vaccines and purchase any of the books on the subject. She suggested homeopathic teething tablets for Clay's teething problem as well. This was my first introduction to homeopathy. The teething tablets were wonderful; they just dissolved on his tongue. When he was beside himself from teething and couldn't sleep, they would settle him down right away. He loved them, and so did I.

She also recommended the book *You Can Heal Your Life* by Louise L. Hay. It was the first book I read that thoroughly discussed the amazing power of forgiveness. I loved it and embraced its philosophies. I had much forgiveness work I needed to do and just thinking the words, "I forgive…" helped. I bought several copies and gave them to people I cared about.

My cousin, a nurse in Ireland, previously warned me about the MMR vaccine when I was pregnant. She told me it caused autism, and none of her children had any of the vaccines. I had asked Clay's pediatrician about it when Clay was two weeks old, and she angrily defended the shots. She was adamant enough about it that I believed her. But the threat of autism still terrified me.

The book I bought on vaccines was written by a doctor, but its ideas seemed too radical for me. It had one chapter on the risks of vaccines, and the rest of the book criticized the medical profession for what seemed like every childhood problem. I have recently read this book again and now know much of what he said was accurate. I just wasn't ready for it when I read it the first time. I now know, however, much more about alternatives to conventional medicine and the risks posed by conventional medicine. It has taken me a long time—and a huge amount of research—to get to this point.

Prior to all of this, I had been a supporter of vaccines. I had a history of bronchitis, and my allergist insisted I get a flu shot every year. When I didn't get one, I would get sick, lose my voice, and end up on steroids and antibiotics to clear up the infection. (I had even been diagnosed with chronic bronchitis.) One episode lasted for four months and several sets of antibiotics before I was given steroids and was finally able to overcome the illness.

I was influenced by my sister as well, whose children were young when the chickenpox vaccine became available. She told me about seeing an entertainer while she was on vacation who warned about the risk of not getting the chickenpox vaccine. He had not given his daughter the vaccine; she got chickenpox, developed meningitis, and almost died. He didn't want anyone else to make the same mistake he had made. It is estimated one in 10,000 children who catch chickenpox will develop meningitis.

This scared me very much. I didn't want my son to die from chickenpox complications. But I was still concerned about the risk of vaccines, so I talked to another pediatrician at our group about it and decided to wait on more shots until I could learn more. The doctor gave me a book to read that *seemed* more balanced. I do not recall the title of the book, and I no longer have it to refer to. But I wouldn't recommend it anyway. It did point out there are risks to vaccines, although it emphasized childhood illnesses can kill your baby. It also talked briefly about the government program that reimburses victims of vaccine damage. I should have seen that as a red flag; however, I didn't. If the vaccines were safe, why on earth would there be a government program set up to give money to people who are harmed by them? It didn't mention the shots are linked to SIDS, seizures, learning disabilities, and the skyrocketing autism rate. It also failed to point out vaccine manufactures are legally protected from lawsuits resulting from adverse vaccine reactions.

I was additionally distracted by the mercury issue. Much of the vaccine debate has focused on thimerisol, a preservative used in vaccines that contains mercury. Many people believe this is the cause of autism. I don't want mercury in a shot given to me or my son, although there appears to be more to it than just the mercury. For instance, flu shots contain mercury; however, they aren't linked to autism. Some shots have been linked to seizures and lifelong epilepsy; others have been linked to SIDS. The MMR seems to be the autistic breaking point for many children. The bottom line is we don't know why these shots permanently damage some children, while other children appear to go unharmed. But they do.

It seemed like the problem was mercury, and therefore mercury-free vaccines were safe. My pediatrician assured me their shots were mercury-free. I later found out many of them were, although not all. Additionally, I would later find out some of the shots given to my son were incubated in chicken eggs, and my son was severely allergic to chicken eggs, which the doctor knew but did not warn me about.

We decided to limit the shots to one per week and go ahead with them. It's a decision I still regret today. Nevertheless, I'm one of the lucky mothers; my son has recovered from the damage caused by the shots. I know of many other people who have not been so fortunate.

13 *Head-Banging*

By the time he was one year old, the doctor finally admitted Clay had allergies and put him on an antihistamine. This was the final straw for Clay. The medicine made him crazy— although it would take me months to figure this out. He was miserable all the time. He started banging his head on window ledges, tables, and even asphalt. Sometimes he would just use his hands to bang his head. His pictures from this time frame made me sad because he had self-inflicted bruises on his forehead.

When I would tell people Clay banged his head, they would say, "All little kids do that." But it didn't feel normal to me. I wondered if the frequency or intensity of Clay's head-banging was worse than other children, because no one else seemed concerned about it. I asked about it at a La Leche League meeting, and a few other mothers had experienced it but they weren't concerned. They suggested I get some good heavy metal head-banging music for my baby. While it was amusing, it was of no help.

It was terrifying to watch my beautiful little baby walk over to the window and bash his head on the sharp ledge. One day his daddy was holding him in the driveway, and I came outside. Clay saw me and wiggled like he wanted down to run to me. He got down and immediately bent over and banged his head on the asphalt. I was beside myself.

He had bruises on his forehead all the time. I even bought a photo editing program so I could remove the bruises on his forehead in my favorite pictures. I talked to the nurse at the pediatrician's office about it, and she was of no help. She kept saying it was behavioral, and he was angry about something. Yes, he was angry—because he was miserable.

Even worse, he would occasionally crawl across the floor on his hands and knees and bizarrely drag his head as he went. It made me crazy; it looked and felt so autistic. I would jump up and pick him up off the ground to keep him from doing it. I just could not watch him do that. It preyed on my darkest autistic fears.

14 *Allergies*

Once Clay was willing to eat solid food around age one, I found out how bad his allergies really were. We determined through a very strict elimination diet Clay was highly allergic to cow's milk, corn, soy, eggs, chocolate, oats, and even table salt. His reaction to allergenic foods was immediate and intense. Cow's milk, including cheese and anything cooked with cow's milk, caused excessive mucous. One night I was feeling weak, and I let him have a bread stick with cheese sauce because he loved cheese. The snot started within minutes. Eggs would cause him to vomit everything up in his stomach. Table salt caused hives; corn, soy, and chocolate caused him to walk on his tiptoes and bang his head on window ledges and the ground. Oats made his face and ears flush.

An elimination diet starts with eating the least statistically allergenic foods, then adding one food at a time, separated by three to seven days, and watching closely for symptoms. Allergy symptoms can be anything that didn't exist before the allergen was introduced, including behaviors like head-banging, foul moods, insomnia, and spinning in circles, to name just a few. Most people think of allergies as mucous and hives, and while they can certainly be an element of allergies, they are by no means the only ones.

Clay was allergic to dust and feathers too. One day my dog had torn up a down pillow, and when my son walked into the room, he started sneezing streams of mucous immediately. When Clay would sneeze, it wasn't the normal dainty achoo I was used to; his sneezes sent streams of yellow and white snot down to his chest, and there were normally three or four back-to-back.

For people like Clay and me who had become allergic to everything, our immune systems were in overdrive all the time, overreacting to anything and everything. As a result, when there was a real threat to the body, such as a virus or bacterial infection, the immune system was so distracted and exhausted it couldn't fight off the real invader. Every little thing made us sick.

I became an expert on allergies. I eventually learned his toe-walking and head-banging were classic signs of allergies, as were his hiccupping in the womb and after birth. Even his early walking at about 10 months was a sign of allergies.

I found and studied the book, *Is This Your Child?* by Doris Rapp, M.D. It's an excellent book that discusses in detail the symptoms of allergies. Many consider it to be the bible on the subject. I recommend it to anyone who is suspicious someone they love has allergies. It is a good introduction to the subject, although many are frightened off by its 600-plus pages. It explains in detail the many and varied symptoms allergies can cause, many of which are behavioral. The other difficulty with this book is it takes a somewhat mainstream approach to treatment. It suggests removing the allergens, shots, antihistamines, and food drops. Food drops function in a similar fashion as allergy shots. They introduce a small amount of the allergen, with the intent of reducing allergic reaction. All of these things can help with the symptoms of allergies, although they don't address the underlying cause of the immune dysfunction.

15 Alternative Care

When Clay was approximately 15 months old, I called a local health food store because I was becoming desperate and the medical community wasn't helping. The first thing the clerk asked about was prescriptions. I said, "Well, he's taking an antihistamine, but that can't be it!" She responded, "That's the first thing I would look at. Did he bang his head before he was taking it?" The answer of course was "no." Unfortunately, she didn't inquire about the shots, because I was still oblivious to their role in Clay's illness.

I called the doctor's office and spoke to the nurse. She said there was no way the antihistamine was causing the head-banging. It had to be a temper tantrum, she insisted. I tried to explain he would be fine one minute and banging his head the next, with no event in between. The only culprit I could identify was the antihistamine. She still said it couldn't be related.

I made an appointment to see the pediatrician and told her the story. She said he didn't have to have the medicine, and if I was concerned, to stop it, which I did. His head-banging became much less frequent, but his allergies persisted. He wasn't really any worse off because the antihistamine didn't seem to improve his allergies anyway.

I went into the health food store to talk to someone in person and to see what kind of remedies they suggested. They recommended Rescue Remedy, which is a liquid Bach flower remedy. It helps with trauma, and I suspected I could get it down Clay. She said if I couldn't get it in his mouth, I could even put it on his skin. It wouldn't work as fast, but it would still help.

She also recommended Calms Forte, a homeopathic blend. I wasn't as sure I would be able to get this down him, but I was willing to try.

16 *The Osteopath*

I originally went to see an osteopath years earlier, at my husband's recommendation, which is a little odd, because I'm the one more interested in alternative care in our family. My husband is an athlete, and knew of this osteopath from a friend. I had hyper-extended my knee snow skiing, and over the next few months, the injury became more of a problem. Eventually the pain was bad enough it was difficult to sleep.

I went to the osteopath prior to seeing a surgeon, and I'm very glad I did. He evaluated my condition and said it was repairable, although it would take some time. He said I also had a lot of small problems, including poor posture from working at a computer; nevertheless, they were all treatable. He was able to completely relieve the pain, swelling, and trauma over the course of six treatments, and I have never had a problem with that knee since.

On another occasion, I had a cyst under my arm. I was very concerned, because I had seen the movie *Terms of Endearment*, and the main character died of cancer that began with a cyst in the underarm. I saw an M.D. about the cyst first, and she said there was nothing she could do. It would just get larger and would have to be removed surgically. I didn't like that idea, so on my next appointment with the osteopath I asked him about it. He said he would look at it at the end of my session, and he was able to completely release it with hands-on manipulation.

He said I would feel crummy for a while because what had been in the cyst was now floating around in my body. He said it had been caused by the aluminum in my antiperspirant, which I eventually gave up and replaced with tea tree oil. This was my first warning about aluminum. It would be many years before I would find out how truly damaging it is. The reason tea tree oil works as a deodorant is it is a natural antimicrobial. The moisture from perspiration isn't what causes the odor; it's the bacteria that grow in the perspiration. The tea tree oil prevents the odor-causing bacteria from growing. I simply put the oil in an atomizer and spray it under my arms like I would an antiperspirant or deodorant. A friend of mine prefers a homemade combination of baking soda and cornstarch.

So here it was years later, and my back was killing me because my sick son insisted on being carried all the time. The small of my back felt like it had been twisted, and it hurt most of the time. I had a knot in my shoulder I had experienced on and off most of my adult life too. The additional stress of carrying my son all the time made it much worse than in the past.

I went to see the osteopath, and he straightened out my back and relieved the pain. He suggested I not carry my son so much, but given Clay's emotional and physical state, it was difficult. I discussed my son's condition with him, and he believed he could help.

The first few visits with Clay were pretty awful. The doctor's office was 45 minutes away, which seemed like an eternity with Clay screaming the whole drive. Then trying to get Clay to lay still on the doctor's table for 30 or so minutes while he cried was heartbreaking. Somehow, I knew this treatment would be worth the heartache.

He said Clay had birth trauma, and his condials were compressed, but it was correctable. It would have been quicker and easier had I taken him immediately following the birth, but it wasn't too late. What the doctor could have corrected in one month would now take several. He wasn't happy about the treatment I received when I had toxemia, particularly the steroid shots.

The mucous in Clay's nose would frequently flow much more after seeing the osteopath, as the passageways were more open; then we would see some improvement. By his fourth visit, he was no longer screaming during the treatment. We started giving him a sucker while he was on the table. At this point in his life, we never let him have sweets, so it was a big treat to him.

Clay still sees the osteopath every four weeks, and he is one of Clay's favorite doctors. Clay comes home from the doctor and says, "Me like me doctor; he fix me nose and me ears."

17 Our First Homeopath

Clay was about a year and a half old when we decided to try a homeopath. In Indiana it can be a challenge to even find one. Our osteopath referred us to someone a colleague recommended, so Clay and I went to see her. She used a machine she pressed on acupuncture points to establish a baseline of our health. One of the first things she asked me about was the baby shots, and whether he had been given any combination shots. I shamefully said yes, with the exception of the MMR. She said, "Thank God."

We both were tested. When she was testing me, she said, "Now don't panic because of these results." I didn't know what the results meant, and I wasn't panicked until she said that. My results were very bad; Clay's, however, were pretty good. "If we can just get his immune system strengthened, he'll be fine," she said.

It was another difficult experience because he had to sit relatively still in my lap for 30 minutes so she could test him. I was the surrogate for him, so she used my acupuncture points, but I still had to hold him. He screamed and cried, and I prayed this would be worth it. It was not.

She gave me about 20 remedies, some of which were liquid herbal and mineral supplements. I could barely choke the liquid ones down. They made my whole body shiver. I never got used to them. She gave Clay about 15 remedies. Luckily they were the little lactose pills that just dissolve on your tongue. Which given his milk allergies, were probably not a good idea, and explains why Clay would later test negative for homeopathics. I had to take a few liquid ones on his behalf; since we were still nursing, it would pass through my breast milk to him. I remember one horrible-tasting one was for reverse polarity, which I now know can be cured easily without supplements. It just has to be released, which I'll explain later.

She forgot to give me something for the head-banging, which frustrated me, because it was my biggest concern. I called afterwards, and she recommended belladonna, a homeopathic remedy.

I didn't see any improvement for either of us, other than I felt like I was doing something. I didn't like going to her office, for a number of reasons. It was in a neighborhood that felt less than safe. Additionally, the first time we were there, the receptionist was loudly complaining about what it was like to be overweight (she was probably 150 plus pounds overweight). The practitioner was also a good 75 pounds overweight. It made me nervous to see a healthcare practitioner who didn't appear healthy, and whose receptionist didn't either.

The homeopath went on and on about the school system, both public and private. She had ended up home-schooling her daughter. She told me a horrible story about her daughter's experience at school, many years prior. I agreed it was a terrifying thing for a child to go through. What I was uncomfortable with was this woman was still angry about it, and projecting that anger out to me. I was just beginning to understand the power of forgiveness, and I knew it wasn't healthy she was still angry enough about it to be venting. She hadn't forgiven them and it showed.

While we were still in her care, I sought out an herbalist who used energy testing to determine what was going on with the body. She indicated Clay had aluminum toxicity and a yeast overgrowth. I had the homeopath test him with the machine, and he tested as having both. She wasn't particularly concerned about either one. She gave him homeopathic remedies for both, although I still saw no improvement in his condition.

Since I was conflicted about this homeopath, I tested it (which I'll explain in the next section), and got a yes. I continued to see her until I found a better practitioner.

18 Energy Testing

About this time I began energy testing everything I put in my mouth or my son's, including foods, drinks, and supplements. It was something I learned to do when I was in college, and played with from time to time although I didn't take it very seriously. At this point in my life, I was pretty desperate, and looking for guidance to make sure the choices I was making were in my son's and my best interest. I didn't want to make another mistake like I did with the shots—just cooperating because someone who seemed knowledgeable told me it was the right thing to do.

I can't overemphasize the importance of testing. There have been so many times when I had a nagging feeling something wasn't right, other than all logic pointed to doing it anyway. When my ego (the logical side) and my intuition are doing battle, testing is the perfect way for me to get to the bottom of the issue. In the past, my ego normally won, and I frequently regretted it. Testing gives me the extra confidence I need to listen to that inner voice or feeling warning me not to do something just because it looks right. I have learned if it doesn't *feel* right, it probably isn't.

One of my red flags is the thought, "I should just get this over with." That was how I felt about the shots and would later feel about other medical interventions. I didn't want to do it, so if I closed my eyes and rushed through it....

There are a lot of theories about these inner voices and feelings. The bottom line for me has been when I ignore them, I regret it. So now I practice listening to them and pray for relief from my ego, which wants to run the show at my expense. The ego is a powerful opponent, and one I continue to do battle with every day.

There are several ways to energy test using the muscles of your own body, or the muscles of someone else's, both of which are called muscle testing, or kinesiology. You can additionally use a pendulum, which is called dowsing. There are whole books written on these subjects, and a great deal of information on the Internet.

Testing gives me the confidence to reclaim my power. Previously, when I had been taking Clay to the pediatrician, I gave her all the power. I let her determine his treatment, even when it didn't feel right and wasn't working. With testing, it helped me to have confidence in myself, to know what was best for my son and not depend on someone else. I found this to be a problem with alternative care as well. If the person had a great deal of conviction he could help, I found myself believing him. Just because someone thinks he can help, does not mean he can.

A good resource on muscle testing is *Your Body Doesn't Lie* by Dr. John Diamond. It is considered by many to be a classic on kinesiology. *The Ultimate Healing System: The Illustrated Guide to Muscle Testing & Nutrition* by Donald Lepore is another good resource on muscle testing. They are both available at Amazon.com.

A good book on using the pendulum is *The Pendulum, the Bible and Your Survival* by Hanna Kroeger, available on line at http://www.hannasherbshop.net. A good website on pendulum use is http://www.lettertorobin.org, as is www.dowsers.org.

To use someone else's muscles, ask the person to hold out his right arm, perpendicular to the ground. He attempts to keep it in place while you push down on it. This establishes a baseline as to how he reacts to the pressure you are exerting. Then ask the person to hold a food, drink, or supplement in the left hand, and push down on the extended right arm again. If the item is not needed by the person's body, if the person is allergic, or if it is bad for the person, the arm will become weak and easier to push down. If his body needs the item, the arm will stay strong or even be stronger. An easy way to demonstrate is with a glass of water and then a cigarette or a canned diet soda. The arm should stay strong for the water and get weak for the cigarette or canned diet soda.

To use your own muscles, the concept is similar. Again, you're looking for a strong or weak response. You can use your middle finger to push down on your index finger: If your index finger gets weak, that's a no; if it stays strong, that's a yes. You even can make an O with your thumb and forefinger, then try to pull it apart with the index finger of your other hand, again looking for a weak or strong response.

You can ask questions of the body. A simple one to start with is "Does this body have a penis?" It's a pretty black-and-white question, so it helps you establish what a weak response and strong response feel like.

To use a pendulum, you need a weight on a string. It can be a paperclip, button, or something pretty. Many new age shops carry lovely pendulums made of semiprecious stones, but to start out, I recommend using something inexpensive. To establish positive and negative, if you're right-handed, hold the pendulum over the middle finger of your left hand. The direction it swings is your positive. To establish your negative, hold the pendulum over the index finger of your left hand, and to establish a neutral, hold it over your thumb. Once you have established negative and positive, simply hold the pendulum over a supplement, inquiring about you, or someone you are testing, and it will swing negative, positive, or neutral.

Energy testing is not perfect; however, I have yet to find a system that *is* perfect. Blood testing and MRIs aren't foolproof, either. With energy testing, if you have expectations or opinions, put them aside before you test, or you may influence the outcome. This is a double-edged sword. Some people doubt the information they receive so much they never become capable testers. To test properly, put aside your ego, wishes, and opinions, and trust in God. He is the one doing the work and providing the answers. In the beginning, it may be beneficial to have someone double-check you. Eventually it will not be necessary because you will gain confidence in the process as you see it work.

Each system of energy testing has advantages and disadvantages. I suggest you try each, and go with the one that works most naturally for you. Muscle testing with someone else's muscles is beneficial because they can see the change in their strength, and it creates emotional buy-in for them. Using your own muscles is quick and can be done privately. Using a pendulum is useful because you can create fan charts where you can quickly go to the area that needs the most attention, or a remedy. A fan chart is simply a chart in the shape of a fan with different information where it fans out, such as ailments or remedies. The pendulum then swings to the most important area.

Just because someone who had a lot of schooling said something was good for my son this *did not mean it was true.* I learned that the hard way. If I was suspicious, I would energy test, and if the answer was no, he didn't take it—I didn't care what the healthcare provider said. The same went for testing. As you'll see later in the book, a couple of doctors wanted to do tests on me and my son that I was guided to refuse. It became very important to me in our recovery that I kept my power and discerned on each issue whether it was in our best interest or not.

19 Our First Alternative Doctor

I told a friend about my experience at the homeopath, and she suggested I see a local doctor who used a lot of alternative treatments, including a machine like I described. I made arrangements to go in by myself before taking Clay. The doctor ordered a lot of tests, a complete blood workup, a computer scan like I had done at the homeopath, and a live cell analysis. I wanted to find out about their allergy testing, and he said the computer would test for all allergies.

Sometime during the treatment he began talking about his own insomnia; it was a chronic problem for him. Again, this concerned me, seeing a healthcare provider who was unable to address his own serious and ongoing condition. How could he help me if he couldn't help himself?

Nevertheless I went ahead and scheduled another computer scan. Prior to doing the scan, I asked the technician about the allergy testing. It was a source of conflict between us. She did not want to do the allergy testing; she said it was important to "establish a baseline first." I said fine, as long as I got the allergy testing. I was still discovering Clay's allergy triggers, and finding one by accident meant his physical and emotional state were going to pay the price of my lack of knowledge. I wanted to see what her allergy testing was like so I could consider it for Clay. We went back and forth on it, and she finally agreed to do as much allergy testing as she could after she established her baseline.

She asked a lot about my medical history, vaccines, bowel movements, aspartame, metal fillings, and a host of other things.

As she was doing my scan, she asked, "What's wrong with your heart?" I thought to myself, "Nothing, until you said that." Her testing method was similar to the homeopath I had seen, but the results looked different. They were still awful, indicating I was very sick. Her testing showed I was allergic to more things than not. I was even sensitive to sea salt. A friend asked, "How can you be allergic to sea salt?" I now know when your body is extremely toxic, you can be reactive to anything.

The doctor ordered a panel of blood tests as well. It needed to be done at a specific chain of laboratory. I drove from my office to the closest lab, which was about 30 minutes away. They couldn't do the panel; only certain branches were authorized. So on another day, I drove to another branch, about 45 minutes away from my office. This time they said they couldn't take a credit card or even cash (I had the exact change). They needed a check, and I don't carry a checkbook. They were closing in 15 minutes for a 90-minute lunch period. I thought I might possibly be able to get to a bank and back before they broke for lunch, because I had no desire to wait around for 90 minutes during their lunch. As I was standing in line at the bank, I thought, "It has been extremely difficult to get this test done. I wonder if I'm supposed to." So I energy tested it, and the answer was no. I turned around and left. I don't know why I wasn't supposed to get the tests. Maybe the protocol the doctor would have prescribed would have been harmful—I don't know—but the universe was certainly trying to tell me not to do it, and I finally understood.

I never ended up taking Clay to see this doctor. I just wasn't comfortable with him, and I lacked confidence he could help me, much less Clay.

20 Aspartame

The woman who did the testing at the doctor's office gave me a book on aspartame, which I read but did not find very helpful. It sounded like a conspiracy theory, making the creators of aspartame sound like evil scientists. Nevertheless it made me wonder, so I energy tested it. I got a definite no, meaning I should not consume it. I tested it for my son, because I had been letting him drink it too, and got another definite no.

I was not happy about this development.

There is a lot of discussion about aspartame and formaldehyde on the Internet and in some alternative health books. The belief is when aspartame reaches body temperature, it turns into formaldehyde. I don't know if that's true, but I do know it is harmful to me and my son because that is how it tests. None of the artificial sweeteners tests positive; they all test negative—including Splenda, which is all the rage now since it is made from sugar. The only thing I have found that tests positive is stevia, which is an herbal sweetener. Even that has to be tested, however, because the manufacturing process can have a negative impact. When I want something sweetened, I prefer raw honey. It tastes the best, and I know it's safe. It tests very positive for me.

What I didn't know about aspartame was I was highly addicted to it. It gave me a rush, a jolt of energy I liked and needed. I really struggled with the decision to give it up. I loved my diet sodas and looked forward to them. I had done the Weight Watchers diet in the past and believed it was a healthy and balanced diet. They allow aspartame, and even let you count sugar-free, caffeine-free drinks as up to one-half of your daily water requirement. I thought it was safe and innocuous, but my energy testing was saying otherwise.

I still remember the last diet soda I had; it was during the Super Bowl with a pizza, one of those lemon-lime ones. I even dreamt about diet soda after I gave it up.

I experienced withdrawal for at least two months. My most noticeable symptoms were my breasts ached, and I would wake up in the middle of the night with a mouth so dry I felt like I had been in the desert. Nothing could quench my thirst. It took me a while to figure out what was causing it, but with the help of an herbalist, I was able to determine it was aspartame withdrawal.

I really regret letting my son have aspartame. He would still consume it if I let him. A friend of ours drinks a lot of diet soda, and I made the mistake of letting Clay have a little recently. He still talks about it, and tells me how much he likes it. I have learned to put up with his tantrums, or he would consume it all the time. It's hard to avoid because it's in foods I would never have expected, like many gums and cough drops—and even flavored waters. I was at a friend's recently and drank some flavored water. It tasted really good, so I looked at the ingredients, and it contained aspartame.

A little friend shared some mints with Clay recently. He had a fit when she took them back. When I looked at the package, they were sugar-free with an artificial sweetener. That explained why he had such a meltdown over them; they gave him a rush or shot of energy, a tiny little high.

Sometimes at a restaurant, when I see a soda being delivered to another table, I still crave one. I will occasionally allow myself a full-calorie caffeine-free soft drink, but I never have diet or caffeine. My body just can't handle it anymore, which is a good thing.

I've had two caffeinated drinks in the past several years. I vividly remember each instance because of the consequences they caused. I was making a two-hour drive and stopped early in the morning to order a cup of hot tea. I was buzzing until 2:00 P.M. At first it was nice to have the jolt to help me make it through the drive. Then the caffeine made my stomach upset and caused my heart to race; I felt like I wanted to run around the room. It wasn't fun anymore. The second occasion I was out to dinner with my husband, and I ordered a cherry-flavored, caramel-colored drink. It tasted so good, I decided to have a second. Boy, did I pay for that. I couldn't sleep that night, and when I finally did, it was restless and anxious. It was not worth it.

This is a good example of how energy testing helped me. I don't know exactly why aspartame is bad for me and my son. But I don't have to wade through the arguments both pro and con because testing answered the complicated question for me very simply. No, my body and my son's body can't handle aspartame. The withdrawal I experienced and the mourning I went through over having to give it up just confirmed to me how deeply addicted I was.

21 The Emotional Healer

The technician at the first alternative doctor's office told me about an emotional healer who was in town for the weekend, and only came occasionally. She suggested I try to see him. I called and made an appointment for both me and my son since he didn't come to town much.

His approach was based on speech, saying things that support your vision and envisioning yourself healthy. It seemed somewhat logical and very positive. I like logical and positive.

I had worn a black outfit with a fairy scene on the front to the appointment. He was critical of it and said I should never wear black, it was a death wish. He asked me, "Would you dress your son in black?" The answer, of course, was no. I went home and got rid of all my black, which was quite a lot.

He believed Clay's illness stemmed from vaccine damage, and suggested I get some remedies it took me a year and a half to find. By the time I found them, Clay didn't need them anymore, thank goodness. He suggested Hanna Kroeger's homeopathic (vibropathic, as she calls it) remedies, which he told me I could order through the health food store where I met him. The store told me they were very hard to get and they would try to order them for me. I was never able to get them through the store. Much later I was able to find Hanna's website, http://www.hannasherbshop.net and order them directly from the source.

The practitioner additionally believed we needed more forgiveness in our family. This is an area I continue to focus on to this day. Forgiveness is always good.

He believed my throat clearing was emotional; I wasn't speaking my mind. That didn't feel right; I have never been accused of not speaking up. I tend to err on the other side, of being too straightforward. I would later discover that even though I had been speaking out about my son's illness, I never felt like I was being heard. So in some respects he was right. However, it was the aluminum that was causing me to be allergic to absolutely everything and creating mucous, resulting in my constant throat clearing—not the fact I wasn't being heard.

I have observed this phenomenon in many practitioners. They believe theirs is the only approach that will work. This man believes everything is caused by our emotions. He was like the guy who only has a hammer, so he thinks everything is a nail. It has been my experience there are many ways to approach the body that are beneficial. There is often an emotional element or lesson in every illness or disease. But speaking up wasn't the lesson I was to learn from our aluminum toxicity. Speaking up more wouldn't have done anything to release the aluminum from my body or to keep me from poisoning myself with it on a daily basis. I needed more than emotional healing to overcome my aluminum and allergies.

He sold me a ton of supplements and tapes. I felt great when I left the appointment, but the simple task of buying the supplements, because there were so many, sucked all my energy away. I felt worse than when I walked in the door.

I had never had so many supplements in my life. It was overwhelming. Taking them every day took 35 minutes. I decided to energy test them, and there were about seven that tested negative. I took them back to the health food store, and the woman tested me with the machine to see if they stressed me. She was stunned to find all the ones I wanted to return tested negative for me. They were things that according to conventional alternative healthcare anyone could take: like Calms Forte, a homeopathic remedy, a flower remedy, and colostrum. Over the course of time, people would keep trying to give me colostrum, and I would continue to test negative for it. I would eventually find out both my son and I were allergic to milk, and colostrum is made from cow's milk, hence, one of the reasons it tested negative.

Since I was continuing to nurse my son, anything that went into my body would affect him. I would always test to make sure everything was positive for both of us. The poor little guy was like a canary in a coal mine. He was our indicator as to whether something was toxic for us. He showed signs of toxicity long before I would.

From an emotional standpoint, I felt like I had made a decision to get better and had a new outlook on life. I would continue to wonder for some time why I wasn't getting better physically.

The technician from the alternative doctor's office additionally tested Clay for allergies, and he was literally allergic to everything she tested.

I stopped seeing the first homeopath and took only a few homeopathic remedies the technician gave me. I was still on all the supplements the emotional healer had given me that I tested positive for, but we still didn't know the underlying cause of all our problems. I did an extensive yeast and parasite cleanse. These stick out in my mind because the remedies were so awful, but I was testing positive for them, so I took them.

An odd symptom I had was a hypersensitive sense of smell. My nose worked better than my beagle's. When I had a cold, before it would develop into bronchitis, I could smell the bacteria and knew where it was heading. I knew someone who used to wash his face with a washcloth that had been wet and sitting out; I could smell the bacteria long before it smelled sour to anyone else. I could only eat meat purchased that day, or again, I could smell the bacteria growth and not be able to eat it. It was such an issue for me I even started writing a fictional book about a woman who had a hypersensitive sense of smell that she used to find and determine the cause of illnesses.

22 Returning From Florida

When Clay was one and one-half years old, we took a vacation to Florida. We stayed at a fun hotel with a lot of entertainment and visited the parks. The weather was nice, and it was a such a nice break. My son wasn't actually happy, but he was much less unhappy. Looking back at the pictures, the only one where he was smiling was the one in the bathtub. At night, when Clay was the most unhappy and difficult to handle, we could go to the hotel. He would walk around, and the employees would play with him and entertain him. It was such a relief.

He got sick with croup over the trip. But even that wasn't that bad. We saw a doctor and told him we didn't want to use antibiotics unless absolutely necessary, and he said it wasn't. He was up all night long one night, but we played in the lobby in our pajamas so my husband could sleep. He had the bad coughing and mucous, but we were pretty used to that by now.

We would go to the park during the day, nap, have dinner, then walk around the hotel at night. He seemed almost content. I was beginning to think maybe things were going to be different.

Then we came home. The very first night, we were back to the slow torture of Mommy and Daddy. He was unhappy all night. All he wanted to do was stand on the bar in the den and pace back and forth. This of course did not make him happy, just less angry. One of us had to stand there, holding on to him every moment so he wouldn't fall or hurt himself. He grunted a lot and cried while he walked across the top of the bar. It was miserable.

A friend of mine with an autistic son called this "stimming on the bar." Stimming is a word used in the autistic community to refer to self-stimulatory behavior that seems to make an autistic child feel better. She was probably right; it probably was stimming, but I hated to hear that term applied to my son.

I was so discouraged. We'd had a whole week that was actually pleasant. We joked about moving to the hotel in Florida so he would be distracted from his misery, and so my husband and I could have a few moments of rest each night.

At home, every evening was a struggle to see what we could do to entertain him so we could maintain our sanity just one more night. We would take him to his grandfather's, the grocery store, or the home improvement store. Things out of the ordinary would buy us a little bit of time where he wasn't crying and miserable. But it wouldn't last. He would get bored, and we'd have to rush him home to avoid the arching back and screaming fit. I would sweat the whole way home trying to keep him happy for the 15 to 20 minutes it took to make the drive.

Whenever he was restrained he was unhappy, and the car seat was one of his least favorite places to be. It was a double-edged sword: We needed it to get him places where he could be briefly distracted, although it was torture getting there because he hated being in it so much. It certainly reduced the places we went, because I just couldn't take the stress of riding with him in the car.

There is a wonderful children's museum about 50 minutes away from where we live. He loved it, but the drive there was horrible. So during the first two and a half years of his life, we only went there once, because Mommy just couldn't take the screaming, crying, and fits he would throw in the car.

23 Narrowly Avoiding the MMR

When my son was about one and a half years old, he was scheduled to go to the pediatrician the next day to have his MMR, and a regular check-up. I had put him down for a nap, and had this incredible, almost irresistible, urge to get on the Internet. I got on, and looked at articles about allergies, because at this point in our lives, his allergies were running his life and mine.

I ran across an article talking about diets to control allergies at a pretty mainstream website, parents.com. The author, Karyn Seroussi discusses her experiences of controlling her son's autistic behaviors like toe-walking (which she points out is very common in autistic children) and dragging his head across the floor, with a diet free of dairy and wheat, commonly known as the gluten-free casein-free diet, or gfcf for short. She would eventually go on to found the Autism Network for Dietary Intervention (ANDI). Toward the end of the article she linked autism, allergies, and the MMR shot together. You can find the article at http://www.parents.com. The article is titled *We Cured Our Son of Autism.* The website for the Autism Network for Dietary Intervention is http://www.autismndi.com/.

I felt like I had been hit by lightning. I knew immediately I was not to ever give my son the MMR. My whole body was electrified with the knowledge that I had been teetering on the edge of disaster, and narrowly escaped by divine intervention.

I had been given a very clear message: if my son were to receive the MMR, with his medical condition, he would become autistic. I could barely sleep that night. If I hadn't found that article on that day, we would have gone to the pediatrician the next day, he would have been given the MMR, and for an already very sick child, it would have pushed him over the cliff.

It reminded me of the story where the holy man is facing a flood. He says to himself, "God will save me!" He is out on the porch, and a truck comes by. "Come with us!" they yell. "No, God will save me!" The water gets higher, he climbs up on his second story balcony, and a boat comes by. "Get in, we can take you to safety," they plead. "No, God will save me," he yells back over the sound of the water. The water rises, and he climbs to the roof. A helicopter comes by. "Grab the ladder; we'll take you to safety!" "No, God will save me," he yells in response. The helicopter leaves and the man drowns. When he gets to heaven, he asks God, "Why didn't You save me?" "I sent you a truck, a boat, and a helicopter. What else did you expect?" God replies.

That story has always made me feel like if something comes up three times, I may not get another chance, and it is probably a message from God. This was my helicopter. I had been warned by my cousin in Ireland when I was five months pregnant, by my mom's friend the acupuncturist, and now I had been divinely inspired to read this article linking allergies, autism, and the MMR. I was not to let Clay have the MMR.

If you would like more information on the vaccine debate, I recommend the book, *Vaccines, Are They Really Safe & Effective?* by Neil Z. Miller. They maintain a website as well, www.Thinktwice.com. Another good website on the effects of vaccines is http://www.unlocking autism.org/, which is the website for Unlocking Autism.

There are risks either way—if you vaccinate or if you don't. Childhood illnesses can be very serious, and in rare cases even cause death. I remember studying up on chicken pox: 1 in 10,000 children will develop meningitis as a result of that disease. Meningitis can be fatal. According to the Department of Health and Human Services 1 in 167 children nationwide is diagnosed with an autism spectrum disorder (ASD), and many people in the autistic community link their children's illness to the shots. I decided the odds were in our favor if we didn't do the shots.

I had never energy tested to see if Clay's body could handle the vaccines, because when I was going through that inner debate, I wasn't energy testing anything. But I did now, and I got a definite no!

As sick as he was, and with all the indicators pointing to autism, the pediatrician would have still given him the MMR, and no doubt, my beautiful little boy would have passed the point of no return. I kept our pediatrician appointment, but of course did not allow that shot.

I was so frustrated. She had been absolutely no help with his lack of development, allergies, and recurring illnesses; she didn't even take any of these issues seriously. My son had been sick for over a year, and she kept telling me it was all normal. But she was always there to try to convince me to give him more shots. She even wanted him to have them when he was sick. It was as if that was all she cared about—that, and feeding him cow's milk. I know this sounds harsh, but in the end, she felt more like a drug pusher than a healthcare provider.

It defies logic. The peds insist the shots are safe; they won't even acknowledge they carry a risk. All medical interventions carry risks, even something as innocuous as aspirin. Why do they turn a blind eye to the risk of vaccines, when there is so much evidence they are harming so many children?

I became obsessed with the link between allergies and autism. The more I read, the more evidence I found the two were related. Most autistic children have several allergies, in particular, milk, corn, soy, eggs, and wheat. My son was allergic to four of the five. Why didn't my pediatrician know about this link? Why wasn't she warning me and taking his allergies more seriously? Why didn't she know that broad spectrum allergies like my son had pointed to a serious underlying immune disorder and a predisposition to autism?

At this point I gave up on pediatric medicine. They hadn't been any help, and I was much more informed on my son's illness than they were. The things they suggested simply made him sicker, and their preoccupation with vaccines at the cost of my son's health was tragic.

I felt lost and alone. My son was very sick, and there wasn't anybody who seemed to be able to help. A close friend asked me, "Have you ever thought about just leaving him alone?" No, I never did. He was miserable, and so was I. Every day felt like just surviving, not living. It was a test of endurance. Why would I settle for a pathetic existence like that?

24 An Herbalist and Aluminum

My mom referred me to a local herbalist, Katherine Lehman, who had apprenticed under a master herbalist. Katherine said Clay had aluminum and yeast. She was the first person to acknowledge how awful he felt. She said, "He's miserable; he can't stand being in his own skin." She was the first practitioner I felt totally comfortable with; I knew she was on the right path, both for herself and for us.

We talked about aluminum a great deal, this was the first I had heard of it. She's the herbalist I mentioned earlier that I saw while I was in the care of the first homeopath. I had heard a lot about mercury, but not aluminum. At the time, I was still drinking out of aluminum cans. As a matter of fact, almost everything I drank came out of a can, including sparkling water.

I was wracked with guilt. I had been poisoning myself and my son with every beverage I consumed. It reminded me of the stories about the Roman soldiers who had been slowly poisoned because their water jugs and water pipes were made of lead. This led to the weakening of the army and their eventual downfall.

I searched the Internet to find information on aluminum poisoning and toxicity, and found the story of a little baby who had died of kidney failure because the mom had eaten 75 antacids every day while she was pregnant, causing aluminum toxicity in the infant and eventual kidney failure. Beyond that, I found some alternative websites that talked about aluminum and how it gets into our bodies, and its link to Alzheimer's, but nothing that indicated how prevalent or serious it could be.

Aluminum is used as a preservative because it prevents the growth of bacteria, so it can be found in small amounts in many things. It is used as an anti-caking agent in things like salt and flour. It is even used as a drying agent in dog food, and if it is less than ½ of 1% it doesn't have to be listed in the ingredients.

I immediately stopped drinking anything out of an aluminum can. We purchased all new cookware that was aluminum-free. I replaced all the table salt in our house with sea salt, which is aluminum-free; we got rid of our conventional baking powder, and bought Rumford baking powder, which is aluminum-free. I used all of our aluminum foil to make animals for my son, and never bought any more.

Shortly after I found out about aluminum, I cooked my son some chicken nuggets I had purchased from a mainstream grocery store. He immediately began banging his head, so I looked at the ingredients, and it actually listed aluminum as an ingredient. I was appalled.

One morning we were out at a restaurant, and my son was playing with the table salt. Before we left the restaurant, his face and neck became covered in hives. We took him home, gave him a bath, and the hives went away. When I asked the herbalist about it, she explained to me how aluminum is used as an anti-caking agent in table salt. I began carrying sea salt in my purse.

On another occasion Katherine scanned me, and said, "I'm not going to tell you everything I found because I don't want to scare you." This of course did just that. She did tell me I had aluminum and yeast, although she didn't tell me what else she found.

She gave me the 15-day yeast diet, which follows. It is much more lenient than any I had seen before. She additionally recommended CanSol, made by Pure Herbs. (Their contact information is in the appendix.) It's an herbal combination that does miraculous things when it comes to yeast. One of the things I liked best about this yeast diet is it allows homemade bread, sweetened with raw honey, and it even allows raw honey to be eaten as a sweetener and to be used in cooking. Most yeast diets restrict you to meat and vegetables, and they are normally at least 30 days. This version is only 15 days long. The only thing is, you can't cheat at all. If you do, you have to start all over again.

Yeast causes the muscles and joints to hurt; and it causes the same symptoms as low blood sugar. It's best to make your own bread while you are on this diet.

15-Day Yeast Diet

- 2 tsp Can-Sol per day made by Pure Herbs.
- 6 L. acidophilus made by Nature's Sunshine.
- Eat no sugar, white flour, vinegar, mushrooms, canned goods or juices.
- Eat fresh fruits only; make your own juice.
- Eat fresh vegetables only, not canned or frozen.
- Raw honey is okay as a sweetener, but it has to be raw, not pasteurized. Most commercial honey is processed. You can tell raw honey because it crystallizes over time. If it does, put the jar in hot water to liquefy it. Do not put it in the microwave.
- Do not use maple syrup as a sweetener.
- Use whole grains; make sure the bread label reads whole wheat flour. If it says wheat flour, enriched wheat, or enriched white flour, do not use it. It is best to make your own bread so you can be sure all the ingredients are safe. Also read the flour labels.
- Whole wheat pasta is okay; so is brown rice.
- No sauces, dressing, condiments, processed cheeses, or processed food of any kind. Most processed foods contain vinegars and chemicals as preservatives.
- Read cheese labels. Make sure no additives or milk sugars have been added.
- Read the milk label; it is best to use lactose-free milk. Lactose is a natural milk sugar. Sugar feeds the yeast.
- Fresh meat is okay, but no processed meats such as bacon, lunch meats, or canned meats.

- It is best to shop the outer perimeter of the supermarket: fruits, vegetables, meat, and eggs.
- Check the label; anything that ends with "ose" is sugar. No Splenda, Aspartame, or other artificial sweetener.

She additionally helped me to identify some common sources of aluminum:

- Aluminum cans
- Aluminum and non-stick cookware
- Anti-caking agent in table sugar and salt
- Baking powder
- Antiperspirant
- Emulsifier in some processed cheese
- Bleaching agent used to whiten flour
- Aluminum foil
- Some toothpaste and cosmetics
- Vaccines
- Cigarette filters
- Aluminum hydroxide
- Antacids, and many other over-the-counter medications
- Synthroid, as well as many other prescription drugs

According to pdrhealth.com, "The major source of aluminum in foods is food additives, such as sodium aluminum phosphates in cake mixes, frozen dough, self-rising flour, and processed cheese, as well as sodium aluminum sulfate in baking powder. Aluminum is found in a number of commercial teas." Their website is: http://www.pdrhealth.com/drug_info/nmdrugprofiles/nutsupdrugs/alu_0020.shtml. It's a mainstream site that tells where some aluminum occurs, nevertheless it goes on to say it's not harmful, which of course it is.

Canada's Healthy Environments and Consumer Safety branch of government states, "The daily intake of aluminum can be greatly increased for individuals consuming maximum recommended doses of aluminum-based over-the-counter drugs such as antacids and buffered acetylsalicylic acid (ASA). The World Health Organization has estimated that individuals who regularly ingest these aluminum-containing pharmaceuticals may have intakes as high as 5 grams per day." The article can currently be found at http://www.hc-sc.gc.ca/ewh-semt/water-eau/drink-potab/aluminum-aluminum_e.html. It has moved in the past, so if you can't find it at this address, just search "daily intake of aluminum" and the article should come up.

Safe aluminum-free alternatives are:

- Cookware made of surgical grade stainless steel
- Iron
- Glass
- Crockery
- Antiperspirants made of rock salt, tea tree oil, green tea, sage, or that say aluminum-free
- Sea salt
- Rumford aluminum-free baking powder

25 Live Cell Analysis

I had a live cell analysis done at the alternative doctor's office. In a live cell analysis, they take one drop of blood and look at it under a highly powered microscope. They can tell you many things about your body and your immune system simply based on this one drop of blood. It sounded weird to me, although I cooperated.

I was surprised at how interesting it was. There were many things wrong that he found through this analysis, the most important of which was there was a large supply of parasitic fungus-based germs in my blood. He said most people would call them yeast, except that was not what they were. It was disgusting, seeing them wriggle through my blood cells, eating them up. He said they were eating my food, and creating waste in my blood.

There were a lot of poorly formed red blood cells, and ghost cells. This provides a breeding ground for the parasitic germs. This was not an area he really focused on; however, later I would learn it was very important. Dead and damaged cells are a breeding ground for infection, bacteria, fungus, and parasites.

He put me on a 30-day sugar-free diet, which basically reduced my diet to meat, nuts, and vegetables. Later on he would tell me the nuts were contributing to the fungus problem. He put me on more supplements too—*like I needed that*. But I energy tested them, and my body did want many of them.

I lost a lot of weight, felt horrible, and when I went back four months later (he said that was how long it would take to get rid of the parasitic germs) to get checked, the parasitic germs were still there. I was so frustrated. I was taking a boatload of herbs, vitamins, minerals, and anti-yeast products, and had made radical changes in my lifestyle. As far as I could tell, nothing was improving. If anything, I felt worse than when I started all of this. My fatigue was constant, I was missing a ton of work, and when I had any free time, all I wanted to do was sleep. It was so depressing. It reminded me of an analogy: If you hold a glass of water up for a minute it seems light, if you hold it up for an hour, your arm begins to hurt; and if you hold it up for a day, you're miserable. In each case, it's the same weight, it's just the longer you hold it, the heavier it seems. I had been holding Clay up for two years.

My son's constant illness, combined with my lack of sleep, was sucking the life out of me. I had given up the stimulants like caffeine and aspartame that had kept me going for the first year and a half of his life. Now I was feeling the full effects of the stress of having a sick child.

26 *ET*

I felt like Elliott in the movie *ET*. In the movie, a little boy discovers and cares for an alien named ET, for the Extra Terrestrial. The little boy, Elliott, and ET develop a link, where Elliot and ET could feel the same things; it's one of the ways they communicate. As ET becomes sicker and sicker from being in an environment that was unhealthy for him, Elliot deteriorates too.

I felt like Clay was ET and I was Elliott. Clay and I were like one being. I was always talking about how *we* felt, how *we* couldn't sleep. I could sense his illness and how awful he felt. I knew when he was exhausted and had to nurse or sleep *right now*. I knew he needed me. I often thought I was the only one in the world who understood him. It made me feel very close to him, and certainly needed, but it was a huge burden.

In the evening, when things were the worst, he would often start screaming and crying for me. My husband would try to help by giving me a break and holding my son against his wishes, but I just couldn't stand it. When he would scream and cry for me, no matter how tired I was or how bad I felt, I absolutely had to be there for him. It was a primitive urge: don't come between me and my sick baby. It caused stress between my husband and me. He saw what taking care of Clay was doing to me, and knew I needed relief, but he couldn't give it to me, because I couldn't let him.

Clay was this little alien creature that no one understood. He couldn't communicate except through me, and I didn't know how to help him but to be there for him. He was in an alien and hostile world with danger at every corner, and getting sicker and sicker as every day went by.

27 *The Allergist*

I sought out an environmental allergist who treated food allergies in hopes he could help my son. He said he would not test a child Clay's age, because it was too traumatic. He suggested I get tested, and use the tools I learned from the process, such as a rotation diet, to treat my son.

I went through the testing. It took a total of 15 hours, and I was quickly convinced having Clay go through it was not a good idea. Instead of the little scratch tests, which are notoriously inaccurate, they used what's called p/n testing, or provocation and neutralization testing. They take varying amounts of the allergen and inject it under the skin, creating a bubble in the flesh. If the bubble gets bigger, you're allergic. If it doesn't, you're not.

They even tested me for chemical allergies, one of which was aspartame. By this time I had given up aspartame, and I thought my system was pretty clear of it. When they tested me for an allergic reaction, I was stunned at my response. My heart raced, I felt like someone had come up behind me and scared me. It was like a mini panic attack. I felt nervous, anxious, and perspired. It was very unpleasant. I realized this rush of adrenaline was what I had been so addicted to when I was drinking diet soda all day long.

It turned out I was allergic to aspartame, every food they tested me for, fungus, all the grasses they tested, and all save for one tree. My allergic reactions were not strong; nevertheless, the fact I was allergic to almost everything was a problem.

The allergist said I had developed leaky gut syndrome, which is when the gut, or intestines, actually become leaky. They are weakened by inflammation, yeast, and trauma. In my case he believed it was probably yeast that had weakened the intestinal walls. When gaps in the intestines develop, particles of food seep out into the bloodstream. The immune system sees the food particle as an invader, something to be attacked, and food allergies develop. In the normal digestive process, a protein is attached to the food while it is being digested that allows the immune system to see the food as a friend. When the food leaks out of the intestines, that protein has not yet been attached.

The allergist said allergies never go away. It is an immune system response just like when we were kids. Once we had chicken pox, our body developed immunity to the illness, so next time we came in contact with it, our body would see the invader and fight it off. For instance, oats had leaked through my intestinal lining, and my body saw it as an invader. It then developed an immune response to oats. Every time I ingested them, my immune system tried to fight the invader off, causing a food allergy to oats. He said it was a myth that you can outgrow allergies. He said all you can do is minimize your reaction to them.

There is a great deal of discussion about leaky gut syndrome in the autistic, allergy, and alternative health community. You can do an Internet search on leaky gut and see many detailed articles on the subject.

The allergist suggested allergy shots, a yeast diet *again*, antifungals, and antihistamines. How many yeast diets was I going to have to suffer through? He said I was actually *allergic* to yeast.

I was able to get the allergy shots without preservatives, so I was willing to cooperate. I was even able to learn how to administer them myself and do them at home, which was a big time and hassle saver.

When I met with the nurse to go over the protocol they were suggesting, she explained they had just discontinued recommending a rotation diet. In some respects I was relieved. I had read about them, and they sounded like a complete hassle. You separate all foods into food families, so anything from a cow, like beef and milk, can only be eaten every four days.

In another respect I was disappointed. I hoped a rotation diet would help my son. I had envisioned the whole family going on it. Because it was so much work, it wouldn't make much sense for just me to do it. I had read about how you color code all the food in your pantry and refrigerator: and blue would be day one, green day two, and so on. Since they didn't believe it was necessary, I didn't bother.

We did implement several allergy management and reduction techniques, such as:

- Removed the carpet in our bedroom and replaced it with hardwood floors, because we were all allergic to dust, and dust mites flourish in carpet.
- Swept or vacuumed the floor and furniture every day.
- Made the dog start sleeping in the laundry room instead of with us.
- Moved all Clay's stuffed animals out of his bedroom.
- Bought special air purifiers for our main living and sleeping quarters.
- Bought a whole-house water purification system, in addition to adding the large bottled water dispensers and bottled water.
- Put special cases on our pillows, mattresses, and box springs that prevent allergens from getting out.
- Washed all our bedding materials each week in hot water to kill the dust mites.
- Stopped wearing perfume and hair spray.
- Switched to allergy-friendly cleaning products.
- Kept all of our windows closed no matter what the weather was like outside.
- Discontinued the use of weed-killing agents, fertilizers, and all chemicals on our lawn.
- Stopped our indoor and outdoor pest control service because they sprayed chemicals each month.
- And of course Clay and I never ate allergenic foods.

I had started down the allergist road with my son in mind. I had no idea I would find myself to be so allergic. I have wondered from time to time why I had to go through all that testing, because I did energy test to find out if I needed to proceed, and the answer was yes. It became apparent to me I needed objective evidence there was something wrong with *my* immune system. It was proof there was something wrong with me too. I just didn't yet know how bad it was, or how to fix it. I had been a sick child as well. Maybe I was born with these problems, and as I grew older, simply compensated for them in other ways. I had never been truly healthy or energetic at any point in my life. That would soon change.

28 Antibiotics

To make matters worse, I developed a pustular rash around my neck and on my chest right after returning from a beach trip. I thought it was an allergic reaction, so I went to see my allergist. He said it was bacterial, something I picked up on my trip, and he prescribed antibiotics. I did not want to take antibiotics because of my yeast problem, so I energy tested them, and the answer was yes. I took them even though I didn't want to. The yeast was quickly out of control, as was my son's. Because he was still breastfeeding, the antibiotics went straight from my breast milk into his system.

The yeast caused nursing to be quite painful, just like it did when he was a newborn.

My allergist prescribed the antifungal, Diflucan. I ended up taking it for four solid weeks before the yeast was under control. A doctor will typically give a dosage of two Diflucan; thirty is almost unheard of.

The antibiotics had started a horrible chain of events for my son. His allergies were even worse than before. He sneezed constantly. He would sleep for two hours at a time, wake up crying and be awake from 20 minutes to a couple of hours.

Clay and I did not get two good nights' sleep in a row. At night and in the mornings I would lay there and listen to his chest and sinuses gurgle with mucous, and pray for relief. When I would put my hand on his back or chest I could feel the vibration and rattling from his labored breathing. I became a walking zombie, and my son was constantly sick and cranky. This went on for over three months.

29 Tubes Are Recommended for Clay's Speech Delay

At 23 months I sought the help of a speech therapist. The evaluation team determined he was communicating at the level of a 14- to 17-month-old. They recommended speech therapy, to which we agreed. They additionally recommended we see an ear, nose, and throat doctor, sometimes called an ENT.

The ENT evaluated Clay, and although I was told by the technician his hearing was within normal parameters, the doctor recommended tubes be put in his ears. He said Clay had mild fluid there, but no ear infection. He wrote a prescription for antibiotics, which I never filled.

I did not want them to put tubes in his ears, so I pushed the doctor on the subject. His response was that when a child has a speech delay, they do whatever they can to correct it, and that included tubes.

It just didn't seem right. Clay had only had a few ear infections, which was a miracle considering the fact he was constantly sick. Plus, they told me his hearing was in the normal range. Yes, there was fluid, but no infection. Tubes seemed awfully radical. It felt like he was recommending them because that was the only thing he knew how to do. At this point in my life, I no longer trusted the medical profession to know what was best for my son. I was suspicious their intervention would just make things worse.

It reminded me of the man who keeps smashing his finger in the door. So he goes to an M.D., who looks at his finger and says, "You need some antibiotics, anti-inflammatories, and a finger brace because an infection has set in." He then goes to a surgeon, and the surgeon says, "It looks like that fingernail has become twisted; it's going to require surgery to fix it." Then the man goes to see an herbalist, and the herbalist says, "I can give you something for the swelling and the infection, however you need to quit smashing your finger in the door."

We got a second opinion on the subject of the tubes from Clay's osteopath. He said no, there is no evidence they work. Our osteopath was already aware of the fluid in his ears, and had been working successfully on keeping them clear. I attribute the lack of ear infections to the talented work of our osteopath.

I energy tested, and got a definite no on the ear tubes.

We chose not to do the tubes and I was relieved. I have since talked to many people who swear by tubes. "My daughter was falling down all the time until she had tubes." "He didn't start talking until he had tubes." It makes me wonder if all these children had the same problem Clay had, and their parents didn't know how to help them, the same way I didn't know.

30 Our Second Alternative Doctor

I found an acupuncturist at an expensive alternative clinic and started seeing her for my fatigue, which had become overwhelming. After several treatments she said, "You're not getting better." I thought to myself, "Why would you be any different? No one else has been able to help." Part of me kept searching for that miracle cure for me and my son. Another part of me was beginning to think it was hopeless, that we would both be sick for the rest of our lives.

There was a doctor at the clinic she thought I might benefit from seeing. I liked the acupuncturist in spite of the lack of results, and was really only seeing the osteopath at this point, so I decided to give her doctor a try. I saw him first, planning to schedule an appointment for Clay if I liked his approach.

He did an extensive background on my medical history, and ordered a boatload of tests. I felt like I gave a gallon of blood. I even had to do a stool analysis, which was a pain—and not in the neck. He said I was an interesting case; you never want to be an *interesting case*. When the lab results came in, he said I won the prize for the worst results he had ever seen. He didn't know how I got out of bed in the morning; he said I had no metabolism. I had a yeast overgrowth, low thyroid, and wasn't producing growth hormone; I had Epstein-Barr, and a host of other weird viruses. He said with all these viruses my immune system should be very elevated, although it was not. Instead, it was depleted. He said I had been sick so long, I was losing the war, which was depressing to hear.

He attempted to determine when and why my illness started. As we discussed my medical history, I told him I had been very sick as a young child. I grew up in a town with a refinery, and it was once in the world record book for having the worst water. I was given multiple vaccines as well when I was five years old because we were going out of the country. He believed those two factors may have been the beginning of my illness. I traveled to Mexico in high school and had gotten quite sick afterwards, which he said was a good indication of parasites. I now also suspect I was born with aluminum toxicity, just as my son was.

He put me on several antifungals, Armour thyroid (which is the preferred choice for those of us who don't like pharmaceuticals), growth hormone, testosterone, ginseng, vitamins and minerals, including several nutritional IVs, probiotics like acidophilus, and a couple of natural sleep aids like melatonin. After several appointments with him, I took 52 pills every day. I remember this number, because a friend of mine was complaining about taking 19 pills a day. I counted mine and I was somewhat stunned to realize how many I was taking. The sad thing about it is, I still felt awful, even though I was choking down all these prescriptions, vitamins, minerals, and herbs each day. Nothing was helping.

One of the IVs was a treatment and a test all in one; some people call it "a challenge." The IV was a chelation treatment. Chelation is a method of drawing metals out of the body. Over the course of the next 24 hours, you collect all your urine, then they test it for toxic metals that the IV pulled out of your body. Chelation is all the rage in the alternative health community. I didn't know at the time there is a growing debate as to how harmful this process is. It's similar to antibiotics; the chelation not only pulls out the bad metals and minerals, it pulls out the good guys too. It is also believed the chelation activates and mobilizes the dangerous metals.

This was the first IV that hurt. From the spot in my arm where they inserted the IV, it hurt all the way down to my finger tips. Plus it made my arm cold from the insertion point down. It was a long hour and a half. Then when they took the IV out, I was so weak I had to go home and lie down for several hours. I was breastfeeding, so I had to pump my breast milk and throw it away because the treatment would pass toxic metals to my son through my breast milk.

One website that discusses some of the risks with chelation is: http://www.dmpsbackfire.com/default.shtml. I now know there are much safer was to remove heavy metals from your body. To remove mercury, simply take vegetable glycerin; to remove aluminum, use the herb bladderwrack; to remove copper use potassium; to remove lead, use horsetail. This was the only IV chelation I agreed to undergo; I don't plan on doing it again.

Aside from the chelation, I liked this doctor's approach overall, so I decided to take Clay in to see him. Clay became hysterical in his office. A lab coat and a doctor were all it took to put him over the edge. Luckily I had someone with me who could at least hold him while I talked to the doctor. She took him out into the waiting room, and I could hear him screaming and crying during most of the appointment. When the doctor saw how panic-stricken Clay was being in a doctor's office he agreed I could come in without him until something should warrant his physical presence.

He did a thorough background of Clay's medical history, and ordered some tests. I came back by myself to get the results. He had several pages of test results, and asked again about his prior treatment. I told him about our experiences with the pediatrician, and how she kept telling me he was fine. "He's far from fine," he responded. "These test results are not good." While it was validating to finally hear an M.D. admit something was wrong, it was also very chilling. The doctor also tested Clay for parasites, and he said just because he didn't find them, didn't mean they weren't there. He said they are very hard to catch in a lab test. He was suspicious both of us had parasites.

We discussed Clay's allergies, head-banging, toe-walking, that he wasn't sleeping, and he wasn't talking. I told him we hadn't been back to see the pediatrician because I didn't want Clay to have the MMR, and I knew she would have a problem with our position.

"A child like Clay who is at risk for autism shouldn't have any vaccines," he commented offhandedly.

The world came to a stop. A doctor had just used the word autism to describe Clay. Yes, he said "at risk," but what did that mean? I had feared and wondered about Clay having, developing, or being diagnosed with autism since he had started banging his head at age one. I had asked the woman who sits for us on Saturday night about it because she owns a daycare center and worked with some autistic children. She said he didn't make the sounds an autistic child makes; but she was concerned about his speech delay.

When I found out about the links between autism, lack of speech, sleep disorders, yeast, and allergies, I became almost obsessed with the subject. My son had all these problems; did that mean he was in the autistic spectrum?

Now I was hearing a doctor tell me my son was *at risk*. "My husband is going to ask me, what makes him at risk for autism?"

"Well, I wouldn't label him like that, but he shares a biomedical spectrum of disorders with the autistic," he responded.

I remember telling my sister what he had said, Clay was "at risk for autism." I couldn't help crying when the words came out of my mouth. She said it was important for him to get diagnosed early so he could get the help he needed when he went to school. We talked about Asperger's, a type of highly functioning autism. She had some direct knowledge of it—both through her profession at an insurance company, and having two friends with Asperger's children.

I did not want Clay to be diagnosed with autism, even if it was *just* Asperger's. I didn't want him going through his whole life with that label, and the burden of being required to tell teachers, counselors, and anyone else who might care for him. I was afraid it would influence their expectations of him and his behavior, and become a self-fulfilling prophecy. A self-fulfilling prophecy is a psychology term; it's when something comes to pass simply because people expected it to happen.

I bought a book on bio-medical treatments of autism. It was pretty creepy. Clay did have a lot in common with the autistic spectrum, and the protocol the doctor recommended was one for autistic children.

He put Clay on a couple of prescription antifungals and some probiotics to treat the yeast. He put him on a liquid multivitamin that is very commonly used for autistic children, and he prescribed growth hormone. Clay was small for his age, and the doctor said that was typical of children with his spectrum of disorders because he wasn't absorbing nutrients from the food he ate.

I tested everything before I gave it to him. He tested positive for the antifungal, and one of the probiotics, but not another, which was packaged in aluminum foil. He also tested negative for the multivitamin, which I was really surprised about. Since the results were unexpected, I asked someone else to double-check me without telling her what I found. She got the same responses I did, so I only gave Clay the items my testing showed me he needed.

31 *The Miracles Start*

At this point in time I had taken Clay to anyone I thought might be able to help. He saw two pediatricians, an osteopath, an ENT and allergist, a naturopath, an emotional healer, a homeopath, an herbalist, a speech therapist, an occupational therapist, and a very expensive doctor who specializes in immune disorders. The osteopath and the herbalist were the only two who seemed to be helping. All the others said they could help, but we didn't see any results.

I had been told Clay and I had aluminum, so I had cut out aluminum from our diets. Everything we knew to be a source of aluminum was removed. I had stopped the contamination, nevertheless I wasn't able to remove the existing levels of aluminum from our bodies and brains. I had no idea how much havoc that was causing in our lives.

With the strict allergy diet, and the removal of incoming aluminum, Clay's head-banging and toe-walking had almost stopped, but he still wasn't speaking. He was cranky, sickly, and not sleeping well.

My mother had an appointment with a master herbalist in northern Indiana, and I decided to go along. Mom, my niece, and I all went together. We made a day of it; we rode up together, visited, and had lunch afterwards. It was the last full day I would spend with my mother before she died.

I didn't take Clay because of the two-hour drive; plus, I never let Clay see a healthcare practitioner I had not seen first. I sat down in the testing chair and told the herbalist I had allergies. He looked in my eyes with a magnifying glass and flashlight, and told me, "You don't have allergies, you have aluminum. You're allergic to everything." I responded,

"Yes, you're right, I am allergic to everything. What can I do about it?" He said, "It's done, it's gone." And he was right. I didn't know what he did, and at this point didn't care.

I felt different immediately. I knew he had cured my allergies. Over the next week and a half, I ate whatever I wanted (aluminum-free, of course) with no problems. Prior to releasing the aluminum, if I ate something I was allergic to, it would cause mucous at the least, and frequently more serious problems, like a whole afternoon of heart palpitations, or fatigue so intense I would have to leave work and lie down. The change was miraculous.

I decided to drive up on a Sunday night with my husband and son in tow, to be there first thing on Monday when they take walk-ins. It was a two-hour drive each way, which at this point in time with my son felt like driving for ten hours. He hated being in the car, and keeping him in his car seat should have been an Olympic event. I just kept telling myself, "This will be worth it…he's going to be cured…this will be worth it."

I had set an appointment when I was there, however he was two months out at that time, and I didn't want my son to have to wait to be cured.

I arrived at the herb shop at 6:20 A.M., and there were 20 cars ahead of me. Mike and Clay came later that morning. I was told it would probably be 1:30 before he could see us, but I knew it would bring Clay's cure, so we waited. It wasn't much fun entertaining a sick and cranky two-year-old all that time. I was so nervous and anxious. I didn't want to leave for fear we would miss our time. I felt like a cat pacing around waiting. Luckily, my husband was patient, and they had some wonderful oatmeal cookies for sale in the shop, which we made our lunch, and eventually our time came.

He asked if this was the first time my son had been to see him, and I said yes. As we suspected, Clay still had aluminum, and he released it on the spot. I asked him if Clay would still be allergic, and he said no. Could he eat eggs and corn? Could I cook with milk? The answer was yes. My heart just flew. I was so grateful. He also checked other things, and worked on him in other ways. At the time I didn't even know what to ask. I was just happy to have the aluminum and allergies gone.

When we left, I was walking on cloud nine. Clay slept well that night, and every night for the next ten nights. He was a new baby, and I was a new person. Sleep deprivation can do nasty things to a family.

Over the course of the following weeks, I slowly introduced foods he had previously been allergic to, always watching for any sign of allergies. I prayed over and over again my fears would not interfere with Clay's healing. One after another, he ate everything with no symptoms. I was so excited; I baked something new every night. To be able to cook with milk and eggs again was wonderful.

My sister would call every day and ask, "How's he doing? What did he eat? Is he having any symptoms?" I would excitedly tell her how wonderfully he was doing. She decided to take her whole family to see the master herbalist too.

The mucous dried up. To see my son without a runny nose was amazing. To hear him sleep and breathe like a normal person, without the constant rattling in his chest and sinuses, was such a relief. And for him to sleep more than two hours at a time, I felt like I had hit the lottery! He said Mommy for the first time about two months after our visit. I couldn't believe my ears. It felt so good. He quickly learned to speak, and within four months, Clay could say almost anything, and was speaking in sentences.

My faith in God was renewed. I thanked Him every day for saving my son and me, and I continue to do so. We had a new life; it was like starting over. Clay was actually healthy. He could eat anything, and not have a reaction. I had been so afraid this day would never come. In the beginning I didn't tell people about Clay's recovery, because it was so far out. I had been taught by my allergist that people can't recover from allergies: "It is an immune response your body never forgets. All you can do is minimize the reactions."

Clay and I were living proof you can be cured, completely and immediately. It was amazing.

There was no more head-banging, no toe-walking, no more stimming on the bar. He was in a good mood almost all of the time, he could ride in the car without freaking out, he stopped getting colds, and his yeast cleared up. Two years of torture had come to an end in one day.

I kept kicking myself because I had known about this herbalist for five months prior to the time my son had seen him. I just couldn't face that two-hour drive with Clay. Plus you had to write to get an appointment. I remember there was a cancellation I heard about, although it was the following day, and I had another appointment already. That was a choice I later came to deeply regret. In my defense, I had seen so many practitioners, and there didn't seem to be anybody who could help. Why would this one be any different? I didn't know anyone who had been cured by him. I just knew he was another practitioner. I certainly didn't understand the immense impact aluminum was having on our health. We went through five months of constant illness and stress that I could have avoided. I have since forgiven myself, because forgiving, even yourself, is an important step in healing.

I had spent so much time, energy, and money trying to get Clay and me healthy. All we were doing was controlling his symptoms, and we weren't even doing a very good job of that. Now we were both cured in moments after a simple unspoken prayer, and no ceremony. I had never heard of such a thing. He didn't even charge us. It was so easy and unspectacular; it was hard to grasp at first. Nevertheless I eventually did.

I struggled to understand the horrible impact aluminum had on our lives. I scoured the Internet, and there was nothing that indicated the devastating effects of aluminum, and the many things it sets your body up for, like cancer. I wondered if what he called aluminum was really mercury, because I had heard and read so much about mercury in the alternative healthcare community. After much research it became apparent to me there simply wasn't anyone out there who knew how destructive aluminum is to the body. Conventional wisdom, even in the alternative health community, only understands a fraction of the harm it does.

Aluminum is one of the worst things you can put in your body. Unfortunately it is everywhere, and very difficult to avoid. Mainstream society doesn't see it as a threat or risk at all. But it is. Even in health food stores many of the crackers, cereals, granola bars, and even toothpaste is packaged in aluminum. It is so well accepted, the packages don't even state aluminum-free or not. The only way to find out if something in a box has an aluminum wrapper inside is to purchase it and look inside, which is an expensive option.

Get rid of your aluminum cookware, aluminum cans, aluminum foil, antiperspirant, toothpaste in aluminum packaging, and any other aluminum you can find. It is inconvenient, your eggs will stick to the pan, and pancakes are very difficult to make, but every time you use aluminum you are poisoning yourself and your loved ones. There is no test except energy testing that accurately measures aluminum. A blood test won't show it because by the time it's a problem it has lodged in the brain and can't be measured. The same goes for hair analysis. You need to know if it's in the brain, and if it is, it is the absolute first thing you need to treat.

If you have broad spectrum allergies, you almost certainly have aluminum. If you have a yeast overgrowth, you have aluminum. If you have Crohn's, you have aluminum. If you have cancer, you have aluminum. You will never be completely healthy with aluminum, and you'll be open to other illnesses until you're clear.

If you don't have someone in your backyard that is schooled on aluminum (which you probably don't), what do you do to get rid of it? The first thing is discontinue your exposure to and consumption of aluminum. Next, release it, which is very simple, and I'll explain it in detail in the next section. Last, energy test to see if it's still there, and if necessary, take the herb bladderwrack, it's a liquid extract. I recommend you get it from Pure Herbs, Ltd. Their contact information is in the appendix. In really severe cases, it sometimes calls for the herb uva ursi, because it is an excellent source of organic aluminum. You can purchase it from either Nature's Sunshine or Pure Herbs, whose contact information is in the appendix.

After removing the aluminum, you may still have to go on a yeast diet, or a cancer diet, or treat the condition, because once those things have been set in motion, they require special treatment. Although if you don't remove the aluminum, you can go on all the yeast diets you want, and you'll never get rid of the imbalance that allows the yeast to overgrow.

I frequently see children with an aluminum nose, which is one that is constantly running, even though there is no cold. The mother has typically become used to it, and says "Don't worry, it's not contagious, it's just allergies." I worry, but not because I'm afraid it's contagious. I'm afraid they will never address the underlying problem of aluminum. It is common for several children in the same family to have aluminum, because they frequently get it from their mother.

32 *Releasing*

So how did the master herbalist cure us? He simply released the aluminum.

There are so many things that can be cured just by releasing them. No herbs, no homeopathics, no exercises—just a prayer of release.

There are three steps in releasing:

- Release
- Reabsorb
- Restore

Those are the three key thoughts and words; the words surrounding them are less important. In the beginning, I would test to see if there was a problem, for instance, "Does Clay have reverse polarity?" If the answer was yes, I would release it saying:

"Jesus, I ask that You release the reverse polarity in Clay's brain, body, and energy field. I ask that You reabsorb his healthy polarity back into his body as God intended it, and I ask that You restore his body to a state of unconditional love and forgiveness as God intended it."

Then I would test to see if he still had reverse polarity, or whatever the problem was originally. In the case of reverse polarity, all it takes is this simple prayer to fix it. The same with aluminum. Just release it, and it's gone. Unfortunately there are things like parasites and yeast that require herbs and diet; however releasing still helps with the symptoms and will speed up the healing process.

When Clay had parasites, I prayed for their release every morning and every evening. It reduced his symptoms, and shortened the length of time I had to give him the herbs once we finally decided to ignore his tantrums during their application.

Now I often abbreviate the prayer to: "Release the aluminum, reabsorb, and restore."

If I have time, I'll say the whole thing, although if I'm out in public, and trying to take care of something quickly, I'll use the abbreviated version. When we talk about this healing technique, we refer to it as releasing, nevertheless we always do all three steps: release, reabsorb, and restore.

You do not need to be with the person to test or release for the person. If you know the person and can picture him in your mind, you can both test and release for them. If you don't know the person, a photograph or handwriting sample will allow you to connect with his energy. Simply lay your hand on the photo or handwriting sample, and you can test and release.

I struggled with releasing. It seemed too easy. I thought the master herbalist had some magical power. In some respects he does, because he has the power of God behind him. Also, he's been doing this for over 20 years; this has greatly enhanced his natural abilities. However he would be the first one to tell you he doesn't do the healing, Jesus does. He is certainly one of the masters, and is highly sensitive to the energies of others. Nevertheless as he explains it, anyone can become sensitive to these energies, like the medicine man who walks out and stands by a plant and says, "This is great medicine."

You can become sensitive to whether an herb, mineral, vitamin, remedy, or food is good for your body or someone else's. I remember the third time I saw the herbalist. I was just beginning to understand his approach; he was trying to find a remedy for my son, who was sitting on my lap. He touched an herb, and my whole body felt exhilaration. He wasn't touching me or my son, but my body knew this was the herb we were looking for. As it turned out, the problem my son was having was one I had passed on to him.

I also struggled with whether releasing would work for me, and my lack of faith interfered with my ability to help myself and others. I was doing battle with my ego. It is constantly in the background whispering in my ear that I am too great or too small for one of God's assignments, which of course, is not true. We are all totally capable of being one of God's tools. When God gives us an assignment, a mission, or a calling, all we have to do is let Him work through us, and His loving power will do great things—things we could never do on our own, like healing.

I was tempted to say all we have to do is get out of His way, although that's not entirely accurate. God is certainly capable of working through us, even when we are not willing. But it has been my experience that when we embrace His gifts, callings, missions, and assignments, we are healed and blessed in the process.

We are not the healers; we're just the ones asking for the healing. At best, we're a conduit for God's healing energy. It is out of our hands whether it takes place or not. Those being healed also have some responsibility. Are they ready to let go of their illness? Do they want to get better? Is being sick meeting some need of theirs? Is it *their* disease; do they hold onto it; is it rare and therefore somehow special? They have to be willing to let go of their illness in order to get better. If they aren't ready, no amount of prayer on my part is going to help them.

We can also become a self-fulfilling prophecy, where we become imprinted with the belief that we are ill when a doctor tells us we have a certain disease or chronic condition. I saw this in my own life. My doctor kept telling me I had Epstein-Barr. I remember the day he told me about the test results. To find out I had this awful virus I had heard so much about, made me so tired I had to go straight home and lie down.

After I recovered from an energy perspective, I continued to see this doctor, expecting him to tell me the test results had changed. Again my ego was at work wanting credit from the doctor for the energy work that had been done, wanting to see test results that backed up the energy work. But they didn't. According to him, I was still testing positive for elevated levels of Epstein-Barr antibodies. It didn't make sense. I felt better than I had in a long time, I was sleeping well, I was taking very few supplements—I was even working out, which six months prior would have been out of the question. I remembered when he originally tested me, he could find no DNA of the virus, so he tested for antibodies instead. He thought I'd had the virus for so long it had settled in my organs.

I had someone double-check the energy testing. No Epstein-Barr was showing up. I had to make the conscious decision to disregard what the doctor was telling me, and further to decide not to let him test me for the virus in the future. I was healthy, and didn't want to become convinced otherwise.

An important factor in releasing is what you release. For instance, when my son was so ill, I tried releasing his allergies, but they were just a symptom of his underlying problem, which was aluminum. Until you get to the real issue, releasing the symptoms helps, but it certainly won't provide a cure. Energy testing is the tool necessary to help you determine what needs to be released.

Sometimes an illness is simply out of our control. I know of a chiropractor whose wife developed cancer. He was able to cure it; nevertheless a month later she died of tuberculosis. He was devastated, but came to understand, it was simply her time. When our time comes, there isn't anything anyone can do about it.

Sometimes people are sick because they are supposed to be; it might be a lesson for them, or for someone in their family. I have been told my son was sick for my benefit. If he had not been so sick, I would never have sought out all the practitioners we saw. I would have continued my unhealthy lifestyle and never been cured myself. I would never have written this book. If Clay hadn't been sick with so many allergies, he would have been given the MMR, and he would probably be autistic today. That would have been a tragedy for my whole family.

I haven't found a perfect way of asking the question, but if I am suspicious I will ask something like, "Is this body allowed to recover from this illness? Is this person capable of recovering given the proper releasing, remedies, and outlook?" Sometimes the answer is no.

33 Imprinting Remedies

An important tool I learned from David, one of the master herbalist's students, is imprinting. It is simple, and so exciting. When you test an herb or remedy, you can see if you can imprint it instead of actually ingesting it. When you imprint, you hold the remedy next to the person's body, and say, "Please imprint, integrate, incorporate _____ a day for _____ days, weeks, months, or years." For instance, I was testing for ACS, an herbal combination that stands for all cell salts. It's made by Pure Herbs and is good for nursing mothers. It's a liquid, so I tested for quantity and duration first. I tested for ¼ teaspoon three times a day for six months. I then tested to see if the whole amount could be imprinted and the answer was yes. So I imprinted it, then I tested to see if the imprint took, and the answer was yes. I further tested to see if there was any value in my taking a further amount orally, and the answer was no.

This is so freeing. I can get the benefit of a bunch of herbs, without taking them. How much easier can it get? It's especially good for children and pets. Getting these herbs down a child or a dog can be challenging, but now I hardly ever have to. I always test to see if I can imprint the remedy and if the whole amount can be imprinted. Sometimes it can't be, but it's always worth asking.

When I started working with imprinting, I wanted to make it more complicated than it actually is. I wanted to say, "Please imprint the energy and beneficial qualities of the herb…," but I tested it and got a no. All I was to say instead was "imprint, integrate, and incorporate." That was it.

I had always wondered why so many people walked out of the master herbalist's office without any supplements. Most practitioners have been thrilled to load me down with a bunch of supplements I didn't want to pay for, much less have to choke down every day. With imprinting, you don't have to pay for them or take them. Really all you need is a good testing kit, which contains small samples of herbs or remedies you use solely for testing. You can make one yourself, and some places sell them. I have a testing kit I just love. It includes some of the top remedies from Pure Herbs, although it is actually sold by Natural Alternatives. Their contact information is in the appendix. It's a great kit, with 64 different liquid herb products. It may seem expensive at its current cost of $245, but it's cheaper than buying all the herbs individually.

I've had questions about how long an imprint will last. Testing will answer that for you. I had one person test for a supplement for three years, and it was possible to imprint the complete amount. This is an unusually long time to have to take something, but the line of work she is in is quite taxing, and it makes her susceptible to things she wouldn't be otherwise.

Not all supplements can be imprinted. For instance, with worms or cancer, you have to take the supplements. I've also found people sometimes have an emotional need to take something. If that is the case, taking the supplement accomplishes something for them. They feel like they are doing something about their condition. It's sort of a security blanket. For instance, I took my father-in-law to see the master herbalist. When we left, he said, "I came all this way and he didn't even give me anything to take!" So you can ask, "Would this person benefit most from taking this supplement orally?" and get a yes or a no, then ask about imprinting.

It feels like there should be more to say about this tool because it is so powerful, effective, and simple. But the fact it is so simple means there isn't.

34 *Release Codes*

Release codes are what they sound like, codes that assist in the release of a condition. I've heard different explanations as to why they work. One says the code gives the body the instructions it needs to heal itself. Any good practitioner will tell you we don't heal the body; we simply give the body what it needs in order to heal itself. One person described it to me by explaining each letter and number has its own geometry and vibration. This geometric vibration can be imprinted onto a person through a release code in a way similar to how one of the homeopathic machines imprints a homeopathic vibration onto a remedy.

I have given some release codes in the appendix, but you can find them yourself. As you are testing, ask if there is a release code that will assist with the particular condition. If the answer is yes, first ask how many characters there are in the code. Then ask for each character whether the first character is alpha or numeric. If it is alpha, ask if it is in the letters A to F. If the answer is no, ask if it is in the letters G to K. If the answer is yes, narrow it down by asking if it is, say, G, and so on until you locate the letter. If it is numeric, ask if it is in the numbers from 1 to 5, and narrow it down from there. If the code is ABC123, simply say, "Release ABC123, reabsorb, and restore."

Sometimes a code can be used for more than one condition; SFQU is used for both aluminum and parasites. This isn't really surprising since they tend to travel together.

These codes can also vary based on the cause of the problem. For instance, I have a friend who is having fertility problems. Her release code is 2GK7M4324. Another woman suffering from infertility may have a different code, since it can be caused by many different things. I've experienced the same thing with high blood pressure; there can be many causes. As a result, there can be many different release codes.

Release codes are very powerful. With some illnesses, such as aluminum, all you need is the release code to get rid of the condition. With other illnesses, such as worms, they can offer great support in the healing process.

It is difficult to communicate their importance until you have worked with them. I suggest you experiment with them and see for yourself how much they assist the body in healing.

35 *Parasites*

After aluminum, the next big thing that surfaced for Clay was parasites. The symptoms were varied, and to me they again looked like autism markers.

He suddenly became very anxious; unexpected or loud noises would elicit a complete meltdown. Out of the blue he was afraid to fly, and he'd been flying since he was three months old. He was terrified the whole time we would be on a plane. He used to love to fly, especially since we almost always traveled with my family and their children, so he had a full-time entertainment committee. Now he was anxious and jumpy from the moment he saw the plane until we were back in the airport.

He began having nightmares and talking in his sleep. The wonderful nights' sleep I had briefly become accustomed to were gone.

He would cover his ears when he was scared, want to be held, and bury his head in my or my husband's chest.

We couldn't take him to the barber anymore because he would become so hysterical. We had never had a problem cutting his hair before. It hadn't seemed to matter to him at all. The only thing he didn't like was the vibrating clippers they use on the back of the neck, so we didn't bother with the back of the neck. Now he wouldn't even let me cut his hair. I had to cut his hair in his sleep, so of course it looked ragamuffin all the time, and I got an endless amount of grief about it.

He also started picking his nose *all the time*, another source of teasing I didn't need.

We had taken him previously to see a live performance of the Wiggles (a children's band) and he loved it. Now, when we took him to see *Bear in the Big Blue House* at the same venue he was terrified. He didn't even want to go into the lighted theater, much less sit through the performance when the lights went down. We would try several other children's shows over the next six months, and his fear just became more intense, and got to the point where we couldn't even get him out of the car.

He became neurotic about the tags in his clothes. We had to cut them out very carefully to make sure there wasn't anything left that would cause them to scratch or rub. Sometimes he would go the whole day refusing to put his shoes on, even though there was nothing wrong with his feet. He just didn't like the way his shoes felt. We said he couldn't go outside unless he put on his shoes, which we were sure would get him to cooperate since he loves to play outside, but he chose staying inside over wearing shoes.

Shoes with shoelaces became a problem because they had to be tied so the laces were perpendicular to his ankle. At first I didn't have any idea what was bothering him. But every time I would put him in his tennis shoes he would begin screaming and crying about the laces being wrong. My sister is the one who told me her son had a similar problem with laces, and she showed me how to tie them so they would be perpendicular. To me it was just another neurotic preoccupation.

We went to a theme park he had enjoyed a year earlier, but now he wouldn't even go on the merry-go-round. The inside rides sent him into a frenzy. He absolutely hated it; I couldn't believe it. What on earth had happened? His allergies were gone, he was 100 times healthier, but now he was becoming neurotic and an emotional wreck. He was absolutely terrified by things he used to love.

He was more sensitive to sound than my beagle. A delivery truck outside when he was inside would frighten him. He could hear me pull in the driveway even though my dog couldn't. He would cover his ears when the vacuum was running and say it hurt his ears. Breakfast with Santa was a nightmare because the ringing bells scared him, and sitting on Santa's lap was out of the question. The TV would sometimes cause him to cover his ears and say it hurt, and we don't listen to the TV loudly. Even the fan in the bathroom bothered him.

The few people I told about his hearing issues thought it was some type of gift, but that's because they didn't have to live with the emotional consequences, fear, and panic noises would cause. One doctor told me maybe Clay could someday work on a submarine listening for bombs. Yuk, like that's a picture I wanted in my head.

We could no longer go through the car wash, because he started screaming as soon as we went in the tunnel. Prior to the parasites he loved the car wash, it has stuffed animals all over, we would point them out and talk about each one, but now he would scream and cry the whole way through.

We took him to see the master herbalist, and he said all the symptoms pointed to parasites (worms in particular), and when he tested him, he tested positive. I had heard of worms of course, but I thought they were something dogs got, and people in Third World countries. How on earth could my son have picked up worms? He explained they were very common, and one of the top things he sees. They are particularly common in children, and the symptoms include:

- Picking of any kind, the nose, ears, bottom
- Nightmares, night terrors, sleep talking
- Nail biting
- Irrational anxiety and fear
- Excess mucous and sinus problems
- Sensory integration issues such as sensitivity to sound and touch, which means issues with the sense of touch
- Sugar cravings
- Hyperactivity
- Weight gain
- Foul mood
- General discomfort
- Lower I.Q.

I would later learn autistic children always test for aluminum, yeast, and worms. Aluminum causes all the allergies, and sets the child up for yeast, which sets them up for worms. The yeast and worms create havoc in the digestive system, making it almost impossible for the body to absorb nutrients from food, hence the starving brain we hear so much about.

Parasites are much more difficult to get rid of than aluminum. It requires four months of herbs, to be dispensed the four days before and after the full moon, a total of eight days each month. The full moon is when the parasites reproduce and become more active. The herbal combination we used is called W-W, 1 teaspoon a day. It contains mugwort, black walnut hulls, male fern, pumpkin seeds, and Cascara Sagrada. It's made by Pure Herbs, whose contact information is in the appendix.

It can be taken internally, which is the most effective method, but it tastes awful, so we applied it externally. To administer it topically, you can put it on the bottom of the feet, or in the belly button. Adults and children can both do this. We made the mistake of getting it in a cut on my son's foot, and he had a complete fit. I have since gotten it in a cut myself, and it does hurt a lot. Make sure the area is free of abrasions, or you may never get your child to cooperate again, which is a problem I faced.

A couple of books on the subject of parasites, their prevalence, and other ways to treat them are *Parasites, the Enemy Within* by Hanna Kroeger, and *The Cure for All Diseases* by Hulda Regehr Clark. Hanna's book was daunting enough, but Hulda's book is even more detailed and discusses the risks hiding almost everywhere. I don't agree with everything Hulda says as far as reaching and maintaining good health; however her description of parasites is quite convincing.

When I began to read about parasites, I found it overwhelming. They are absolutely everywhere, and almost impossible to avoid. I stay away from some obvious risks like sushi and sausage, but beyond that, I occasionally test for parasites, and when necessary, treat them. My husband takes W-W every month during the full moon to make sure he is clear.

It took us about ten months to get rid of Clay's parasites. Part of the delay was I didn't know what was wrong. Then when I did find out, getting the W-W on him became a huge battle every night after I got it in a cut. I didn't know what I had done wrong, so I didn't even get it rinsed off right away.

I tried cheating by using a prescription worm medication. I tested it, and he tested positive for it, but it didn't completely get rid of the worms.

So we went back to the W-W, but this time we put it on his belly button. It was still quite an ordeal, and he cried the whole time, but I knew he wasn't going to get better until we conquered the parasites, so we suffered through his fits.

There is also frequently a problem with polarity when parasites are present. Reverse polarity, or an imbalance in your polarity, means the magnetic field in and around your body is either going in the opposite direction than it is supposed to be, or there is some type of imbalance in the magnetic field. Reverse polarity will make you feel crazy, but it is very easy to fix. All you have to do is release it, reabsorb the healthy polarity, and restore. I once took an absolutely awful remedy for reverse polarity, when all I had to do was release it, but I didn't know that then.

After Clay was clear of parasites, his symptoms were immediately gone; the nose picking, nightmares, fear of flying, being easily startled by sounds, and tactile issues. The next time we took a trip it was the first time in nine months he wasn't afraid to fly. During the parasite infestation, the whole time we were in the air he would say, "No high, no high," and be jumpy and anxious, and inclined to cry. What a relief to have him free of those little monsters. We even took him to see a live performance recently, and he enjoyed it once again.

I have been asked why parasites cause a fear of flying. The simple answer is we don't know. What I can tell you is worms, or parasites, are a dark force. In some ways it is worse than aluminum or yeast because there is another intelligence present. When you work on someone with worms, sometimes you can even feel another negative life-form.

We could now take him to the barber, with very little fuss, and get him a decent haircut. No more struggling in the dark with a flashlight and a pair of scissors.

All of his sensory integration issues were caused by parasites. There are dedicated therapies and whole books written on sensory integration disorders, and all my son needed was a parasite cleanse.

A sudden loud noise will still scare him, although it will not cause a complete meltdown. He rarely holds his ears these days, and only occasionally has nightmares.

I was stunned at what a different boy he was once he was clear of parasites. I remembered I had also been afraid of flying, but early on in my introduction to alternative healthcare I had done an extensive parasite cleanse myself. I am no longer afraid of flying. What a relief. I remember I had even seen a hypnotist about it, and it didn't help. It was those nasty little parasites.

36 Speech and Music Therapy

During my son's illness we also used some mainstream therapies. Clay began speech therapy shortly before he was cured of aluminum and his allergies. I found the speech therapy the most helpful to me, because the therapist taught me how to interact with my son when he couldn't speak, and when he was learning to talk. I was making some basic mistakes such as anticipating his needs so he didn't have to verbalize, or pretending I understood him when he babbled nonsense. She also taught me to always give him choices, so as he made mental selections, he would eventually make verbal selections. His progress after he was cured was fabulous, because he had just been cured of his underlying problem, which was aluminum.

Before we knew about and tackled the parasites we also used music therapy. Music therapy is very popular in the autistic community. I've read many families have really found it helpful. We did not.

It was a four-month process, where he had to listen to music every single morning through a headset. Because he was having sensory issues he didn't like the headset, and sitting still has never been one of his better qualities, especially when he had parasites.

We started with only one minute of the music therapy, and it created sleep disturbances for him, so we eventually had to bump it down to 30 seconds. It was hard to believe it was even having an impact. We never got past 60 seconds, because every time we increased it, he would have side effects. He frequently didn't like the music, and I found it to be a burden without any obvious benefit. Four months of music every day, even on vacation, and I couldn't see any improvement. On top of that, it was very expensive.

Clay's sensory issues were caused by parasites. Once the parasites were gone, the sensory issues were gone.

Looking at my son now, you would never know he was sick, and you certainly wouldn't suspect autism. He can say anything he wants, he's healthy, he interacts well with adults and children. His sensory issues are gone, he can eat anything without symptoms, he's happy 95 percent of the time, he doesn't climb on the bar anymore, he doesn't bang his head or toe-walk, he'll let us wipe his nose and cut his hair (sometimes), and he can ride in the car without having a fit. If he does get upset about something, he normally bounces back. It used to be if he got upset about something the whole evening would be ruined, because he would never get back in a decent mood.

Our son is like a different child. Our lives are normal, no longer dictated by the health, mood, and tantrums of our son. We sleep well, eat a normal diet, and we thank God every day for these huge blessings that so many people take for granted.

37 Why Did Clay Recover When Other Children Don't?

During his illness, all I saw were his similarities to the autistic spectrum. Now that he has recovered, I've had the time to do much more reading about autism. I also have several friends with autistic children. I now see how much Clay *did not* share with the autistic spectrum. He always liked to be held, he would smile when he was happy (even though that didn't seem very often to us), he would make eye contact most of the time, and he interacted with children and adults. Even at his sickest, he would still communicate, even though it was nonverbal.

All of this became very important to me because I have since tried to help several autistic children recover the same way Clay did. Unfortunately, they haven't. They went to the same herbalist Clay went to, they all had aluminum, and one of them had parasites, however they are all still autistic. What's the difference? First of all, if Clay was autistic it was mild. He carried many of the markers, and I was certainly afraid he was autistic but his case was not severe.

He also didn't have the MMR, and I've been told by two different people I trust very much that had he received the MMR, he would have become autistic. One was a spiritual mentor of mine, and another was an accomplished herbalist. We will never know for sure if that is true, because I will never take the risk and let him have the shot. But even if he were to have the shot today, he is a different child than he was at 15 months when the shot was due. He is healthy now, and could possibly throw off the harmful effects of the MMR. It's just not a risk I'm willing to take.

Clay had also been seeing a very talented osteopath for a full year by the time his aluminum was released. This put him in a much better position to recover.

38 I'm Finally Fertile at Age 43

After Clay and I recovered, I asked about my fertility. One factor was the aluminum. When you have aluminum, it frequently causes dropped organs below the solar plexus. This drops the uterus and makes it almost impossible to become pregnant. I also had calcified ovaries. Calcification is fairly common, and you can find it in any organ. It occurs when there is trauma to an organ; the body sends calcium, a natural healer, to the area. The difficulty is then the calcium becomes hard, hardening and calcifying the organ.

To fix dropped organs caused by aluminum, simply release the aluminum and the dropped organs, then reabsorb, and restore. The same with calcification: release the calcification, reabsorb the healthy organ, and restore. It's simple.

Immediately after this energy work was completed, I started having regular menstrual cycles, like clockwork every 28 days. I don't think I had ever had regular, much less clockwork cycles. I remember on two separate occasions going four months without menstruating. It was common for the length between my cycles to be almost two months.

After getting a clean bill of health on an energy level for my fertility I saw my fertility doctor. I didn't want to go through the emotional roller coaster of trying to conceive if I wasn't ovulating. He didn't think there was much of a chance I would become pregnant, nevertheless he was willing to cooperate with my request. The first thing he did was check my FSH or follicle stimulating hormone level on day three of my cycle. The test was perfectly normal.

I continued taking my Armour thyroid, one grain a day, because I continued to test positive for it. I include this piece of information because the immune specialist I saw believes low thyroid is the single biggest factor in infertility. But taking thyroid had no impact on my cycle, while the energy work did.

I then used an ovulation predictor kit to see when I was ovulating, and I went in for one ultrasound to see if I was producing satisfactory follicles. In the past, even using their biggest gun, micro-dose Lupron, I only produced tiny follicles. On this occasion, there was a normal-sized follicle in my right ovary; however the one in my left ovary was too small. This was all drug- and hormone-free. I would later discover my left ovary was calcified again, which accounts for the small follicle.

I became pregnant that month. I was ecstatic. To become pregnant, with no hormones, no shots, and no in vitro fertilization was such a blessing and such a miracle. I was finally fertile and pregnant at age 43.

I had spent a great deal of time, energy, and money for the years of fertility treatment prior to conceiving our son Clay. I had taken so many drugs, months and months of hormone shots, the short needles, the long needles, shots in the stomach, thighs, and buttocks. I had numerous blood tests, ultrasounds, and repeated disappointments when my cycle started each month. This time I was free to enjoy my pregnancy without the tether of fertility treatment. It was wonderful.

A few people tried to minimize the miracle, and say, "It's common for people with fertility problems to become pregnant after the first pregnancy." That is not true. You may have heard of someone who was lucky enough to become pregnant after fertility problems; however, that does not mean it is common. In fact, it is very rare.

There are also different levels of fertility problems. The person they heard of may have just had to take hormone pills in order to become pregnant; there are also different levels of injectable hormones. I don't personally know anyone who became pregnant without drugs after fertility treatment except me. I've *heard* stories about people who became pregnant after adopting or a successful fertility treatment. I do however personally know several women who never were able to become pregnant, even with the best fertility treatment—and huge investments of money, time, and emotional energy.

It made me feel sad when people minimized the wondrous nature of my pregnancy, but they were speaking out of ignorance. I also prayed these naysayers would not diminish my faith in God and the miracle pregnancy He gave me.

At the time I became pregnant, Clay was still in the midst of his parasites and his hypersensitive hearing. This is relevant because the people who provide the music therapy have a theory that the ultrasounds may be a contributing factor to hypersensitive hearing. As a result, I refused to have further ultrasounds. The nurse at the fertility doctor was stunned I wouldn't have more ultrasounds and said, "How do you monitor the pregnancy?" "The old fashioned way I guess—with a stethoscope," I responded.

My O.B. was my next naysayer. She insisted on reading the statistics to me stating how likely I was to have a Down syndrome baby: 1 in 32 at my age. She then went on to tell me if there was something really wrong I would simply miscarry. She desperately wanted to do an ultrasound, which I did not want. She then offered to do a blood test called the alpha pheta protein that further measures my risk for a Downs baby. I told her I did not want the test done, for a lot of reasons. The test is notoriously inaccurate. Even if it were accurate, and told me for sure the baby was Downs, I would not terminate the pregnancy, so why add the stress? They did the test anyway, against my wishes, when they were drawing blood for another matter, and called me with the results. I felt like they were trying to brainwash me into believing I was going to have a Downs baby.

The results were statistically better than the norm for my age, as though that were supposed to be some kind of relief. Well it wasn't. I was not happy with my O.B. and her office, and I told them so. They had just put another rock of doubt on my back.

My O.B. was also concerned about preeclampsia during this pregnancy and so was I, because I personally know two women who develop this condition during each pregnancy. My O.B. kept watching for it, although based on my previous experience, I knew I would have to depend on alternative health to prevent and treat it if necessary.

I energy tested for magnesium on a regular basis, since even my O.B. admitted this is an underlying cause of preeclampsia. It varied during my pregnancy; sometimes I tested for as many as six magnesium tablets a day, and sometimes none. I would test once a week and set out that week's pills. I had also taken magnesium at the herbalist's suggestion to help with the fungus-based parasites that had been identified in the live cell analysis. He said my body wasn't forming red blood cells properly, and the poorly formed red blood cells were a breeding ground for parasites. I think I took nine a day for four months prior to becoming pregnant. So this by itself may have fixed my magnesium imbalance.

I noticed when I had constipation, I tested positive for more magnesium, which makes sense, because magnesium relieves constipation. The one thing that frightened me about taking magnesium is if you take too much it can cause loose bowel movements or even diarrhea. I worried about the baby and meconium, which is baby's first bowel movement. This is the greenish substance that builds up in the bowels of a growing fetus and is normally discharged shortly after birth. However, occasionally it can be discharged while the baby is in the womb, and that is very dangerous. If you are pregnant and taking magnesium, make sure you discuss this with your midwife, or O.B. I know I haven't been particularly supportive of M.D.s in this book, but there is a time and a place for them; pregnancy can be one of them. But as always, don't give away your power. Make sure you agree with whatever it is they are suggesting. You are an intelligent person. You know more about living with your body than they do. When in doubt, tell them you want a second opinion, or just stall so you have time to go to the library or online to do some research.

I also stayed in the constant care of my D.O. (osteopath). There were a lot of things he tended to while I was pregnant. He said the preeclampsia required support for my liver and kidneys. This helped to prevent the swelling that precedes the condition.

Then I started having headaches, which scared me because that is often a sign of preeclampsia. In one instance, it was a side effect from extensive dental work I had done. My D.O. said sitting in the dental chair with my mouth open like that for four hours caused all kinds of problems, with the symptom being headaches. He recommended when I have to have such dental work done I come and see him immediately following.

I frequently had difficulty breathing, one time to the point where it almost felt like it would bring on a panic attack. It made me think this must be what it feels like to be asthmatic. I found it very scary. The osteopath said mine was actually the opposite of asthma. The constriction on my diaphragm made it difficult for me to breathe in air, whereas an asthmatic can't expel air. He would relieve the pressure around my diaphragm so I could take in air more easily. It was quite a relief.

Then of course, there was the tiny bladder that comes with the last trimester of pregnancy. He acknowledged this is simply part of being pregnant, however he was able to relieve some of the pressure, which was also causing some swelling in my left foot.

The herbalist worked on several things while I was pregnant. He said preeclampsia is caused by the spleen not dumping uric acid, and you can test for it with safflowers. He tested me several times, and it was always a negative. He also said morning sickness was caused by the spleen, so whenever I would get morning sickness, I would test for problems there, and release whatever I found. I did begin having a little bit of swelling in my feet. He said it was the spleen being calcified, released it, and the swelling stopped.

At one point during the pregnancy, my breasts became extremely tender and painful. He said my ovaries were calcified, released it, and the pain improved a great deal. I was still having a shooting pain on the outside of my left breast, and when I tested it, I found the mammary glands had become calcified and constricted. When I released it, the pain was gone. It was so gratifying to be able to tend to my own healthcare needs, and it was so simple. The hardest part was finding out what the exact problem was, and frequently even *that* was easy.

I also tested for calcification in my diaphragm, lungs, and milk ducts at different times, and when they tested positive, releasing the calcification provided great relief.

My fatigue returned during the pregnancy, and the herbalist told me my thyroid had become calcified. This would cause the baby to be too big. The O.B. had already told me he was measuring a little big for his age. He released it, and I felt somewhat better, other than a little low on energy. One of the complicating factors for me was I was working on this book, and I would frequently wake up in the middle of the night with a thought, and not be able to go back to sleep until I had written it down. Luckily I was able to nap in the afternoons, and I did so almost every day.

The master herbalist checked the baby, and said he was healthy and free of Down syndrome. I had, of course, tested several times to see if the baby was healthy, and the answer was always yes. But I didn't think I was particularly objective, and was afraid my wishful thinking might be affecting the test results.

In the final stages of my pregnancy, I was finally at peace that the baby was healthy. I prayed about it almost every day, asking the Lord that the baby be healthy physically, mentally, spiritually, and emotionally.

39 The Happy Ending

My second son, Asher, was born healthy: no Downs, no aluminum, no parasites. The only thing was a little damage to the 24th chromosome, which was easily fixable. Chromosome damage is fairly common; I always check for it when I start working with someone. It can either be inherited, or caused by a prolonged condition. You simply release it.

We are not doing the baby shots, so his chances of staying healthy are much greater than for my first son, Clay. Asher is rarely colicky; and growing like a weed.

Clay continues to be healthy. We've had a second bout of parasites and are treating them with W-W. His polarity flipped at the same time, as polarity and parasites often come together. He has recovered emotionally as well physically. We are still very close; I suspect we always will be. It feels like we went through the war together. While he used to be totally dependent on me, he now has a wonderful relationship with his father, a best friend, and several other children he enjoys playing with. He still comes to me when he's tired or hurt, which feels normal. The first time he chose to go play with a little friend over spending time with me, I was stunned. It was so unfamiliar. But he really enjoyed it, and I'm happy to see him blooming.

I'm healthy, with nothing interesting to write about me, which is good.

My husband, like my son, fights with parasites and reverse polarity. So it's something I check on a regular basis for both of them.

Before we found the right energy and herbal medicine, Clay and I were both so sick. I was afraid he was autistic; he had many of the characteristics of an autistic child. I was infertile, allergic to everything, and it was a Herculean task to drag myself out of bed every morning.

Once we found out what was wrong with Clay and with me it was so simple to fix and treat. With Clay it was aluminum that caused all of his allergies, his inability to speak, many of his autistic behaviors, and his yeast. The parasites caused all of his sensory integration issues.

Aluminum was the underlying cause of all my problems too, causing broad spectrum allergies that made me incredibly susceptible to illness and caused a host of symptoms like mucous and intense fatigue. It was also the underlying cause of my infertility.

Aluminum is so easy to fix. All you have to do is release it, and stop putting it in your body. Even if you don't believe in the spiritual aspect of releasing, you can cure it with the herb bladderwrack and sometimes uva ursi.

Parasites are more difficult because it takes four months of herbal treatment. But, that is better than a lifetime of sensory issues, as well as all the other issues that parasites cause. Aluminum, yeast, reverse polarity, and parasites are often found at the same time, or one right after the other. So if you have one, keep your eye out for the rest. They can all be serious if left untreated. Aluminum sets you up for many serious diseases such as cancer, Crohn's, and Alzheimer's. Both yeast and parasites can look just like cancer to modern medicine.

My son's story and mine both have a happy ending. He was born sick, and I didn't know it. Then he became more sick with each vaccine he received—and because we continued to contaminate ourselves with aluminum. Once the aluminum and the shots were released, he made a miraculous recovery.

I was also sick and didn't really know it because I had become used to it. Plus I was consuming things I thought were safe, such as aspartame. When I quit doing that my true lack of energy surfaced and I crashed with a thud. But after a little bit of energy work and some herbs, I was finally fertile for the first time in my life at age 43. What a blessing.

This is a perfect place to end this book. Things are good in my life. I hope this book helps you with yours. I will likely write additional books as I learn of new approaches to holistic health. I already have one in mind. But for now you've heard the most pertinent parts of our stories. We were very sick; modern medicine wasn't helping. In fact, it was making it worse. But a prayer and some herbs cured us both.

AFTERWORD

Circulating a manuscript to get input is a normal part of the publishing process. As I circulated this manuscript, I got some questions I hope to answer for the reader.

What about the master herbalist? Who is he? What's his background, is he a holy man, is he a preacher, is he a doctor, where did he study, how did he learn to work miracles?

What I can tell you about him is he's a humble man, who tries to keep his ego out of his work. He wants God to get the credit for the healing, not him. He already has more business than he needs or maybe even wants. He wants others to learn how to do healing work themselves. That is one of the reasons I wrote this book—so you, the reader, can learn to diagnose and treat yourself, your family, and friends. You can even become a practitioner.

He is a family man who has a deep faith in God. He has spent a tremendous amount of time studying herbs and prayer, and now he has students like me taking his work out into the world.

I decided after much deliberation to leave his name out of this book. When I asked him if I could use his name, he said it would be fine if I left it out. I would later find out that publicity has in the past caused problems for him. I was disappointed in this, because I wanted him to get credit for the great work he has done. But throughout history, those who discovered and brought forth new truths have been ridiculed and persecuted. So in this instance, he discovered this healing art, and I am simply one of those bringing it forth on his behalf.

To support the effort of bringing his research and work forth, I have started writing a second book that gives even more treatment protocols for other illnesses and diseases. In the meantime, if you're sick, learn to energy test. Anyone can do it. Time and practice do improve your accuracy and results as it does with any endeavour. If you're having trouble, pray about it. Ask God for help. You may be called to muscle test, or use a pendulum. God will show you your way. Listen to Him, not others. This has been hard for me, on several levels. I wanted to be able to muscle test, because many of the people I study with muscle test. I wanted to fit in. In some circles in the alternative health community it's cool to muscle test, but not to use a pendulum. And of course in some circles it is exactly the opposite.

I have always been able to use the pendulum accurately and successfully. Muscle testing has often eluded me. I can do the big and obvious stuff for demonstration purposes. If I have people hold their arm out to establish a baseline, then have them hold a cigarette, or a canned diet soda, of course their arm gets weak. But to determine which of several helpful herbs is best for a person, I have to go to the pendulum. There are levels of good, just like there are levels of bad. I can easily determine this with a pendulum. It swings much more forcefully with the proper herb or remedy. It is a weaker swing if the one I'm testing will help, but there's a better option within my reach.

I have prayed and prayed about muscle testing. The message I finally understood was, I have the gift of an accurate pendulum. I am not accurate with muscle testing, so I should not pursue it. I should focus on the gifts I have instead of wishing I had someone else's. So I have finally dropped the issue and I now focus on accurate pendulum work.

The next frustration I had was I was getting different answers than my mentor. This was really a problem for me. Sometimes I would find things he didn't and sometimes it was the other way around. I discussed it with one of his students, who said, "If you find something he doesn't, release it."

One day I was observing a student work on a woman who had damage to her vocal chords. She was a singer, and I was getting that she had parasites. I suggested the student check for parasites, and he got a no. So the master herbalist said to check to see if she had parasites in the vocal chords and the answer was yes, which makes sense. Whenever there is damaged tissue, there is a good chance there will be parasites and bacteria—just like when there is a dead animal by the side of the road, there are normally some type of parasites eating it. But the real point is, the way you ask the question affects your answer. He was focusing on her body as a whole when he asked about parasites. I was focusing on her vocal chords. She did not have systemic parasites, but they were present in her vocal chords. So, we were both right.

On another occasion, I had tested a friend of mine with cancer, and he was testing positive for parasites. The master herbalist said my friend did not have worms. I asked about it, and he said, "Cancer is parasitic." Also, we all have parasites. There are good parasites in our digestive system that assist with our digestion; and a lack of them causes a yeast overgrowth. These beneficial bacteria, or friendly parasites, are essential to good health. So now I either ask, "Does this person have worms?" or I test for W-W. If they need W-W, they have worms or harmful parasites.

I've seen the same thing with yeast. Everybody has yeast. It is only a problem if it is an overgrowth. So now I either ask, "Is there a yeast overgrowth?" or I test for Can-Sol. If they are testing positive for Can-Sol, they have a yeast overgrowth.

Then sometimes I just get different answers. This was really frustrating in the beginning. I wanted to get the exact same answers as my mentor. To me that would have proved I knew what I was doing. But that was not to be the case. For instance, I was having symptoms of worms, such as rectal itching, painful bowel movements, and excessive gas. My testing showed I needed W-W. I asked the master herbalist about it, and he said it was my spleen. So I quit taking the W-W. Then I developed blood in my stool and wrote to the master herbalist. He said it was worms. I was disappointed with myself because I had known I had worms, but not trusted myself. I was looking outside of myself for the answers.

Once again, I was giving my power away to somebody else, just like I did with the pediatrician, only this time it felt more comfortable because it was an herbalist. But it really wasn't any different. I was still letting someone else make a decision for me when on at least one level,

I knew what I needed. I just didn't believe my testing and myself. I trusted the master herbalist more than what God was revealing to me.

Well, I have learned my lesson. I need to believe, trust, and act on what God shows me. I don't know why God reveals things differently to other people, but He does. It is my job to listen to what He tells me.

One practitioner said it's as though we are all looking at someone who is standing in the center of the room. We all see the same person, but from different angles, and would describe what we see differently.

I've been aluminum-free for two years now. But I recently discovered a layer of yeast in my bowels that is just now surfacing. I had conquered the systemic yeast a long time ago, but this little section was hiding under the surface. There are many layers of healing, and while I've knocked out the big guys, there are still small things to work on. This section of yeast surfaced about the same time the worms appeared.

So does that mean the worms were there previously, like the yeast? Possibly they were dormant. I don't know. But worms and yeast often travel together. If you have a yeast overgrowth, your digestive system is weakened. This sets you up for worms. Worms are almost impossible to avoid. They aren't just in undercooked meat. The ova or eggs can be on the top of a carrot. That is one of the reasons it is so important to wash your produce. Then of course there are pets, which make it difficult to avoid worms.

Once I started treating my yeast overgrowth and worms I was finally able to take off the four pounds I'd been fighting with for ten months. Then I went on to take off another 11 pounds on top of that. Of course there is the added bonus that my scalp doesn't itch, and I don't have to wash my hair every day. Also my bowels move every time I eat, and they are pain free and comfortable. The constant gas has almost disappeared. I'm also less anxious. Worms cause a lot of irrational anxiety.

One of the reasons I wrote this book is when Clay and I were really sick, there was no book out there explaining the miraculous art of releasing. I didn't know how to get healthy and looked for two years before I found the answer. There are no downsides to releasing, no side effects. It is so simple many people have trouble grasping it. It is easier to believe you need to go see a miracle worker than it is to believe God gave you the ability to heal yourself. But He did.

With herbs, there can be side effects. There are two books I particularly like on herbs. They are *Herbal Extracts, Build Better Health with Liquid Herbs* by Dr. A.B. Howard, and the accompanying supplement. Both can be purchased from Pure Herbs (see Appendix II for contact information). There is also the herbal *PDR*. It's not my favorite, but it is a resource. It is particularly beneficial if you are taking prescription drugs; you need to make sure there are no contraindications.

If this book has not given you what you need to energy test and release on your own, then I apologize, because that was certainly my intent. If you feel a need to see someone who practices this art, write to me, and I can refer you to a student of the master herbalist. My recommendation is, don't go as a patient, but as an apprentice. Learn how to test and release. If you struggle with it, go back and read those sections again. If they seem simple, they are, because God does it, not us. Everything is easy for Him. Put your faith in God, and you can be a tool for His healing. If you trust in God to work through you, you will be able to participate in miraculous things.

If you have a story you would like to share, please write to me at Joyous Messenger, Inc., 12160 East 216th Street, Noblesville, IN 46062. I plan on writing other books on the subject, and a compilation of healing stories would be very uplifting.

MY PRAYER FOR THIS BOOK

"God almighty, I ask that this book reach people. I pray it communicates the message of how damaging aluminum, yeast, and parasites are to our health, both physical and emotional.

"I pray it warns parents of the immense danger that lurks in each and every vaccine. Lord, please open the minds of all involved to the risk of vaccine damage.

"I pray people are empowered by this book. Please help them come away from this book seeing, feeling, and knowing how easy it is to become healthy with the tools you have given all of us.

"Lord, I pray the appendix grows to meet the specific needs of all those who read this book and want your help. Please guide me to answers for them.

"Lord, I ask that this book lift the spirits of those who read it. While our journey was a painful one, and it seemed like an eternity at the time, it was only two years. Many families face a lifetime of autism or serious illness. You saved us, and showed us how to become and stay healthy. I thank You for this most generous gift. I request I successfully share it with all who are interested.

"God, I ask that we find a natural cure to all cases of autism, no matter how severe.

"Thank You so much God, for the opportunity, blessing, and gift of writing this book. I pray I am forever Your joyous messenger and humble servant."

Tenna Merchent

APPENDIX I

These remedies came from my studies with the master herbalist and his students. It will be very helpful if you learn to energy test in order to use these notes. But if all else fails, you can treat based on symptoms. When the notes say check xyz that means test to see if either that herb is helpful or if there is a problem in that organ or area. If the herb is helpful, then test to see how much per day is needed, and for how many weeks or months.

Don't be surprised if the number of capsules, drops, tablespoons, or teaspoons is high. Start by asking 1–5?; 6–10?; and so on, then narrow it down from there. The great thing about herbs is you take a lot of them for a brief period of time, say four months, then you're done. The organ is healed, or the problem is gone. It's great.

Also, all herbs and supplements are not the same. Vitamin E, when tested, will vary greatly. Some vitamins don't even test as vitamin E. Two companies we know are high quality are Nature's Sunshine and Pure Herbs. I also like Standard Process. For homeopathic remedies, Hylands is my favorite. If you choose to use any other supplement companies please test to make sure the supplement will actually do what it is supposed to do. It's worthwhile to point out, just because you get it at a health food store, does not mean it is healthy or even safe.

For supplements that are a combination, such as W-W, I've listed their contents, in case they should no longer be available, then you would at least know what herbs are involved.

Do not expect what you read below to match with what you will find in the books of modern medicine. But if you do have one of these conditions, you can expect these remedies to support your recovery.

Here is an example of how to check for things:

Acid Reflux

Check gallbladder and emotional. In this case, check to see if the gallbladder is causing the acid reflux. If the answer is yes, check further. Is it gall stones, is it calcified, is there a virus, is it bacterial? If the answer is yes to any of these, release what you found and test to see if it still needs herbs or if it will resolve itself. If the answer is no, and you check emotional, and the answer is yes, ask, is it anger, resentment, abandonment, low self-esteem, fear, or grief. Release whatever you find and ask if it will now resolve itself.

Acne

Check for a hormone imbalance, the thymus, toxic aluminum, and trauma, release SFQU and check for HSN-W by Nature's Sunshine.

ADD

Check Focus Attention Powder by Nature's Sunshine. This formula contains Bacopa moniera leaves, ginkgo leaf, and grape seed extract. Check to see if the thymus is low. Release the baby shots. Check for yeast.

Adrenals

For support check for HY-A by Nature's Sunshine, it has licorice root, dandelion, and horseradish. Check for early childhood trauma.

AIDS

Check for IVY-D by Pure Herbs, which contains iris (Wild Blue Iris), violet (spring violet), and yarrow, if testing positive, start testing at 40 drops three times per day, which is ½ teaspoon. Check Target Endurance by Nature's Sunshine. Release VNJ and CTX.

Allergies

Check for aluminum with bladderwrack by Pure Herbs. If negative, look for a disruption, parasites, something in the brain. Anything that interferes with the brain causes hypersensitivity. Look for a brain allergy. It could even be dried blood in the brain. Check for B-Complex and Four both by Nature's Sunshine. Check for genetic allergies. If it is a genetic allergy, release it. Check for emotionally charged memories, from being told they were allergic to something and release.

ALS

Can be caused by an overabundance of vitamin F. In this disease, the central nervous system is being attacked. Release ODT-9. Also check for mercury, and if positive, use vegetable glycerin to remove mercury. If there are silver fillings, investigate whether they should be removed by a metal-free dentist that specializes in mercury removal. When removing silver fillings the dentist needs to use a rubber dam in the patient's mouth, as well as an oxygen mask over the patient's nose. If the doctor is not skilled in this matter, seek out one that is.

Aluminum

Test for it with bladderwrack. Release SFQU, and the aluminum. Check for uva ursi by Nature's Sunshine or Pure Herbs.

Anemia

Check the spleen and the twelfth chromosome.

Anorexia

Check for bipolar disorder with cudweed by Pure Herbs. Release the bipolar then check to see if cudweed is still needed.

Anxiety

Anxiety is frequently caused by worms and harmful parasites. Release parasites with SFQU. The herbal remedy for parasites is W-W by Pure Herbs. Take one teaspoon starting four days before the full moon, and finishing four days after the full moon for four months. W-W contains mugwort, black walnut hulls, male fern, pumpkin seeds, and Cascara Sagrada. It can be taken internally, rubbed on the feet, or put in the belly button. It also helps to use clove the remaining days of the month. I have also had success taking it every day for thirty days.

If parasites continue to be a problem after completing the W-W, try olive leaf by either Nature's Sunshine or Pure Herbs. If you have pets, worm them too.

You can also use the lime you get at a garden shop on your yard to kill the ova. This is toxic, so don't let pets or children go in the yard until after you have watered or there has been a storm.

Check for bipolar with cudweed by Pure Herbs, and release. Check to see if the adrenals are weak, if so test for Pantothenic Acid, B5, or Adrenal Support, all by Nature's Sunshine.

Asthma

Asthma is often a depleted adrenal. Check for aluminum with bladderwrack and release. Release chemicals out of the bronchials. Check for pantothenic acid and a breathing formula (such as LH or ALJ from Nature's

Sunshine or AB from Pure Herbs). Also see an osteopath who does cranio-sacral work. There is a pathology associated with asthma that can be corrected by a trained osteopath. They can relieve the pressure around the lungs so the asthmatic can take air in. Check for fear and release.

Astigmatisms

Check vitamin A and D. Check to see if you need to release the silver nitrate drops they used to give babies at birth.

Athlete's Foot

Check for a lack of zinc.

Autism

Release the aluminum. Then work on healing the gut. This requires Can-Sol by Pure Herbs, two teaspoons a day for at least one month, possibly for as long as six months. Pair that with Nature's Sunshine acidophilus to get the good bacteria back in the digestive system. At the same time give one teaspoon of W-W every day for at least a month. The W-W will get rid of most of the parasites. At the same time you can use skullcap to balance the zinc-to-copper ratio. Once the person is no longer testing positive for Can-Sol and W-W, use Olive Leaf Extract every day for at least a month to get the last few remaining parasites.

After the olive leaf, you can begin testing for B.&N.C.-W by Pure Herbs (stands for Brain & Nerve Cocktail), broad bean, catnip, cudweed, food enzymes, Heavy Metal Detox by Nature's Sunshine, lecithin, papaya mint, PDA (Protein Digestive Aid) by Nature's Sunshine, trace minerals, wormseed, and zinc. The wormseed is particularly good for children with super-sensitive hearing. You may need to adjust their herbs as often as every week. When Clay and I were sick, the supplements we tested for changed every day.

Check to see if folic acid was too low while in vitro. If so, release it. Also check for and release genetically low folic acid. Then check to make sure they can absorb folic acid.

If the child is experiencing constipation, test for Cascera Sagrada, vitamin C, and magnesium. Release OKCDM. Release the stimming behaviors. Check for wormseed if there is ear batting. This can also be caused by the adrenals, so release the adrenals. Test for birth trauma and release. Release the lack of communication within the brain. Visualize the brain communicating effectively, picture it in six different sections, then visualize each section communicating and connecting with all the other sections.

Bee Sting Allergies

Check the adrenals.

Bell's Palsy

Check B-complex.

Bipolar

Check for bipolar with cudweed, then simply release bipolar. Check to see if the person needs the herb cudweed and check the hypothalamus and thalamus. Bipolar can be caused by a head injury, release OTE and QGM.

Bladder, Small

For frequent urination, check for cytomegolovirus with yarrow. Check for aluminum with the herb bladderwrack and dropped organs, which are caused by aluminum (see aluminum). Release the aluminum and the dropped organs.

Bleeding

To stop abnormal bleeding check for capsicum.

Blood Clots

Use magnesium to prevent blood clots. Aspirin is buffered with magnesium, which is why it helps prevent heart attacks. Women use three times more magnesium than calcium, magnesium strengthens bones, some calcium weakens bones. To dissolve blood clots use arnica, it can even be applied topically.

Calcification

Calcification occurs anytime there is stress in an area. Calcium will deposit in the stressed organ and can even cause stones. Calcium is the body's natural healer, and when there is trauma or stress, calcium will accumulate, and then can harden, causing problems. Just release the calcification and stones in that organ if necessary. If the stones won't release, test for S.D.-R. from Pure Herbs. If you find calcification in an organ, it is likely to reoccur, so keep an eye out.

Cancer

Check for parasites and yeast, then check for a protein overgrowth and the diet listed below. The protein overgrowth is the real cancer. You can have cancer without aluminum, so check for aluminum. Cancer is a pancreatic enzyme deficiency, caused by aluminum. If it is prostate cancer, also check for S.D.-R. by Pure Herbs.

Nutrition Balance for Protein Overgrowth
- Do not use a microwave.
- Instead of sugar use raw honey. Make sure it is not pasteurized; it must say raw on the label.
- Instead of salt use Bragg Liquid Aminos.
- For nine weeks take:
  One teaspoon Red Clover Blend by Pure Herbs
  One teaspoon whole apricots
  Six food enzymes by Nature's Sunshine
  Six parsley by Nature's Sunshine
  Six pau d'arco by Nature's Sunshine
- At the same time, you need to follow this diet for 4 months:
  Make fresh daily: one qt. carrot and celery juice, mixed
- For four months:
  Eat only fresh fruits and vegetables, whole grains, nuts (especially almonds), legumes, real butter, and cottage cheese (no salt).
  Omit all animal protein, eggs, cheese and other dairy products, sugar, salt, white flour, peanuts.

Canker Sores

Check for L-lysine by Nature's Sunshine, and release OQUR.

Compulsive Behavior

Check for bipolar with cudweed, if positive release and see if cudweed is still required. Check for low blood sugar, and if it is low, check the 21st chromosome for damage. Check the 12th chromosome for damage, and if positive, release.

Constipation

Check for magnesium, check the gallbladder, and check for parasites (see parasites).

Crohn's

Check for the following:
- Aluminum, and release
- Parasites (see parasites)
- A paralyzed and calcified colon
- Intestinal Soothe and Build by Nature's Sunshine; start testing at six daily for four months

• Target Endurance by Nature's Sunshine if the case is quite advanced

Cytomegolovirus

Check with yarrow, if positive release and see if yarrow is still required. Release QPDR.

Dead Tissue

To remove dead tissue use Sundew by Pure Herbs.

Diabetes

Check for interference in the pancreas such as parasites (see section on parasites) or stress. Prescription insulin has side effects, it can cause blocked arteries, and it keeps the pancreas from working. One of the reasons diabetics get heavy is they develop an insulin resistance. Once the pancreas begins working, the blood sugar will start to drop. A diet of raw fruit, vegetables, and lots of protein can be very beneficial to a diabetic.

Down Syndrome

Check for missing 20th and 13th chromosome.

Dyslexia

Check for:
- Baby shots; you may have to release them several times
- Focus Attention by Nature's Sunshine
- Kelp
- Aluminum
- Genetics, cranial fault, pressure on the brain, and vegetable glycerin

Eczema, Cradle Cap, or Rash

Check for the herb chickweed. You can take the pills, make a tea, or rub the affected area. Check for spleen damage, it can be genetic or calcified. Release MIP.

Emphysema

Check for damage to the 26th chromosome, release OCL; check for elecampane by Pure Herbs. If it is a child, the herb can be painted on the feet.

Endometriosis

Check with yarrow to confirm that it is endometriosis. Endometriosis can be caused by the cytomegalovirus, which grows in the body under stressful conditions. Release QPDR and the cytomegalovirus. Check to see if they need to take yarrow and FCS II made by Nature's Sunshine. Check for the quantity of each as well as duration. Start by checking nine of each for four months.

Fibromyalgia
Check for
- The cytomegolovirus in the kidneys
- Aluminum with bladderwrack by Pure Herbs
- Yeast with Can-Sol by Pure Herbs
- Parasites with W-W by Pure Herbs
- Thyroid problems

Flu
To prevent, take 1 to 2 una de gato (Cat's Claw) per day. If they already have it, check for yarrow, catnip, C.C.E.-W, and Herbal Adjustment by Pure Herbs when nothing else works. You can put the Herbal Adjustment on the bottom of the feet if necessary.

Frostbite
To get rid of frostbite, take horsetail by Nature's Sunshine.

Glaucoma
Check for a lack of manganese. If positive, release it, then test to see if they need to take manganese.

Gout
Check for:
- Damage to the 12th chromosome, if positive, release it
- Damage to the spleen, and the spleen's inability to dump uric acid
- B6 by Nature's Sunshine, PDA by Nature's Sunshine, safflowers by either Nature's Sunshine or Pure Herbs, and uva ursi by Nature's Sunshine

Hay Fever
Check for Four by Nature's Sunshine. This formula contains blessed thistle herb, catnip herb, pleurisy root, and yerba santa herb. Also check for B-complex by Nature's Sunshine. This formula contains rutin, wheat germ, rose hips concentrate, and acerola fruit extract.

Herpes
Check for L-lysine and black walnut, both by Nature's Sunshine.

Infertility

Check for aluminum and dropped organs. If present, release both. Check for calcification of all female organs, ovaries, fallopian tubes, and uterus. Check for yeast and a tilted pelvis. Check blue vervain, red rasberry, yarrow, and FCS II, all by Nature's Sunshine.

Lead Poisoning

Check for horsetail by either Nature's Sunshine or Pure Herbs and Knitbone by Nature's Sunshine.

Lupus

- Lupus is a form of rheumatoid arthritis.
- Check for damage to the 18th chromosome. Modern medicine has numbered chromosomes as it saw fit. The 18th chromosome, energetically, carries the marker for lupus. Release the damaged 18th chromosome.
- Check for yeast with Can-Sol.
- Check for a calcium and sodium deficiency, which if it's really lupus, will be there.
- Release toxic calcium and toxic sodium. The release code for lupus is QSFS.
- You need to get the calcium out of the organs, and back into the body fluids. The herbs that will be necessary are burdock, calcium, parsley, yucca, and una de gato. Burdock is a natural liver cleanser; it releases swelling and hard spots in the liver. Parsley provides diuretic properties, as well as rebuilds weak muscles and iron-poor blood. Parsley provides an easily digested source of vegetable iron as well as B-vitamins. Yucca is an anti-inflammatory and a natural steroid. Una de gato, or Cat's Claw, is used in South America to cure rheumatoid arthritis, a condition caused when the autoimmune system attacks the body. It is an excellent immune builder and is used for cancer widely in Europe and South America, where they believe any cancer is curable.
- Homemade celery juice will help a lot, although many people are frightened off by the strong taste. You can put apple juice or anything else in it that will make it taste good.
- As the recovery progresses, other things are likely to surface such as yeast, parasites (maybe more than once) and heavy metals.

Mastitis

Check the ovaries and uterus for calcification, trauma, and stones. Check the milk ducts and nipple for trauma and calcification. Check for lecithin. Check for overabundant milk supply.

Mercury

To remove mercury, check for vegetable glycerin.

Menopause

Check for S.M.&W.-S by Pure Herbs. Take one teaspoon a day for between six months to a year.

Migraines

Check for gallstones and the gallbladder. Check liver cleanser and lecithin both by Nature's Sunshine. Check to see if it is hormonal; check for blue vervain by either Nature's Sunshine or Pure Herbs.

Morning Sickness

Morning sickness can be caused by the gallbladder; check for an imbalance or virus. Check for ginger.

MS

Do not use a microwave. Check for:

- Mercury poisoning with vegetable glycerin. In this case you have to get the metal fillings out right away. Make sure you go to a dentist who uses a rubber dam and oxygen while removing the metal. Find a dentist who specializes in non-metal dentistry. Use vegetable glycerin to remove the mercury from the body once the metal fillings are gone.
- Research Formula by Pure Herbs
- A grain-free, sugar-free diet
- Lecithin

Nail Biting

Check for parasites with W-W (see parasites).

Night Terrors

Check for parasites with W-W (see parasites). Check for bipolar with cudweed (see bipolar).

Organ Transplant

To support organ transplants, check for elecampane by Pure Herbs.

Parasites

Release parasites with SFQU. The herbal remedy for parasites is W-W by Pure Herbs. It contains mugwort, black walnut hulls, male fern, pumpkin seeds, and Cascara Sagrada. It can be taken internally, rubbed on feet, or even put in the belly button. Use one teaspoon for eight consecutive days starting four days before the full moon, and finishing four days after the full moon for four months. The full moon is when parasites reproduce. I have also had success taking W-W every day for one month.

It also helps to use clove the remaining days of the month, which can also be applied topically.

Dead tissue is a breeding ground for parasites. Check sundew because it removes dead tissue. More parasites surface after dead tissue has been digested, because it uses up their nest.

Check for reverse polarity because it often accompanies parasites. After completing the W-W, check for olive leaf from either Nature's Sunshine or Pure Herbs to clean up any remaining parasites.

Polyps

Check for bayberry to dissolve them.

Poison Ivy

To relieve the symptoms of poison ivy apply jewel weed, either in its natural state, or from Pure Herbs. A truly healthy person should not get poison ivy. It means they have an underlying toxicity, such as chemicals, viruses, or they are not eliminating waste properly. Also check for BP-X by Nature's Sunshine, it supports blood and kidney health as well as healthy bowel function and digestion, which in turn supports blood quality. BP-X contains: burdock root, pau d'arco bark, red clover tops, sarsaparilla root, yellow dock root, dandelion root, buckthorn bark, Cascara Sagrada bark, yarrow flowers, Oregon grape root, and prickly ash bark.

Pregnancy

Check Feverfew from either Nature's Sunshine or Pure Herbs. If she hits on it, she is not releasing petosin. Release this inability to release petosin. Check for Red Raspberry by either Nature's Sunshine or Pure Herbs as it supports a healthy pregnancy. During childbirth, once the petosin has been released (when the pain starts down the back in labor) take Blue Vervain by Nature's Sunshine and birth should take place within the hour.

Prostate

To support prostate health, check for PS2 by Nature's Sunshine. It contains: pumkin seeds, saw palmetto, licorice root, black cohosh root, gotu kola aerial parts, capsicum fruit, golden seal root, ginger root, dong quai root, lobelia aerial parts, and kelp plant.

Psoriasis

Check for HSN-W by either Nature's Sunshine or Pure Herbs. It contains dulse, horsetail, rosemary and sage. This combination provides a significant amount of organic silicon, which is required for healthy skin. Check to make sure silicon is being absorbed, and for damage to the 14th chromosome. Watch the sugar during this process as it feeds the fungus that aggravates the condition.

Receding Gums

This can be caused by fluoride in toothpaste and by plaque getting in between the teeth and gums. Use T.G. & P.-W (Pure Herbs) to remove plaque from under the gum line and to get the gums to grow back. T.G. & P.-W contains a blend of white oak bark, mullein, marshmallow, mugwort, indian tobacco, skullcap, knitbone, black walnut hulls, gravel root, red root, and myrrh. All you need to do is swish it around the gum line; it is not necessary to swallow it. Use this product every day until the condition is improved.

Shingles

Apply peppermint oil lightly, then apple cider vinegar; this will kill the pain.

Schizophrenia

Check for bipolar with cudweed by Pure Herbs. Release the bipolar and see if the cudweed is still needed.

Sinus Problems

Check for aluminum, which causes allergies. Check for Four by Nature's Sunshine, check for vitamin C. Four contains blessed thistle, catnip, pleurisy root, and yerba santa. Check for parasites with W-W by Pure Herbs; check for yeast with Can-Sol by Pure Herbs.

Skin Cracking

Check for zinc by Nature's Sunshine. Make sure the body is absorbing it, and if not release the inability to absorb zinc.

Staph

Check for PLS 2 by Nature's Sunshine. It contains slippery elm bark, marshmallow root, golden seal root, and fenugreek seed.

Sunburn

If someone is getting a sunburn too easily, check to make sure he is releasing beta-carotene, that there is not an imbalance or toxicity in the silicon.

Stroke

To prevent stroke, take capsicum by Nature's Sunshine.

Teething

Release BZ48 and check to see if the baby needs one teaspoon of liquid calcium per day. Check to make sure he is absorbing calcium.

Toenail Fungus

To release, put greasewood extract by Pure Herbs on top and it will kill it. It may take ten weeks or more of daily application to completely remove the fungus.

Toxemia, Preeclampsia

Check for safflowers by either Nature's Sunshine or Pure Herbs. It can be caused by the spleen and inability to dump uric acid. As a result, the kidney isn't able to function.

Warts

Warts can be caused by a zinc deficiency, so check zinc by Nature's Sunshine. To remove them use the milk from milk weeds, it can be done without scarring or pain.

Water

We should all drink one-half our body weight in ounces of water per day. So if you weigh 140 pounds, you need to drink 70 ounces per day. It is also important to drink water that is free of toxins, and that has a proper ph balance of about 7.0. You can get litmus testing paper at the health food store to test your water.

Yeast

Check for aluminum with bladderwrack and for yeast with Can-Sol, made by Pure Herbs. With yeast there is always aluminum. You will never get rid of the yeast without getting rid of the aluminum. If the person tests positive for

Can-Sol, use the diet below. You can't cheat on the yeast diet at all; even one time means you have to start over.

15-day yeast nutrition

- 2 teaspoons Can-Sol made by Pure Herbs. This formula contains purple loosestrife, white pond lily, and greasewood.
- 6 L.Acidophilus.
- Eat no sugar, white flour, vinegar, mushrooms, canned goods or juices.
- Fresh fruits only; make your own juice.
- Fresh vegetables only.
- Raw honey is okay as a sweetener, but it has to be raw, not pasteurized. Most commercial honey is processed. You can tell raw honey because it crystallizes over time. If so, put the jar in hot water to liquefy it. Do not put it in a microwave.
- Do not use maple syrup as a sweetener.
- Use whole grains. Make sure the bread label reads whole wheat flour. If it says wheat flour, enriched wheat, or enriched white flour, do not use it. It really is best to make your own bread so you can be sure all the ingredients are safe. Also read the flour labels.
- Whole wheat pasta and brown rice are okay.
- No sauces, dressing, condiments, processed cheeses, or processed food of any kind. Most processed foods contain vinegars and chemicals as preservatives.
- Read cheese labels. Make sure no additives or milk sugars have been added.
- Read the milk label; it is best to use lactose-free milk. Lactose is a natural milk sugar. Sugar feeds the yeast.
- Fresh meat is okay, but no processed meats such as bacon, lunch meats, or canned meats.
- It's best to shop the outer perimeter of the supermarket for fresh fruits, vegetables, meat, and eggs.
- Check the label. Anything that ends with -ose means sugar. Use no Splenda, Aspartame, or other artificial sweeteners.

APPENDIX II

Contact information of companies suggested in this book.

Natural Alternatives contact information:
Natural Alternatives
1151 SW 30th Street • Palm City Fl 34990
877-242-2632
www.naturalhealthbalance.com

Nature's Sunshine contact information:
Nature's Sunshine
P. O. Box 19005 • Provo UT 84605
www.naturessunshine.com
800-223-8225
You can purchase their products from some health food stores and practitioners. To purchase directly from the company you must sign up to be a distributor, and there is a nominal fee.

Pure Herbs contact information:
Pure Herbs, Ltd.
33410 Sterling Pond Blvd. • Sterling Heights, MI 48312
586-446-8200 or (800) 860-4372
www.pureherbs.com
Pure Herbs specializes in liquid herbal extracts. You can purchase Pure Herbs products from some health food stores and practitioners. To purchase directly from them you have to sign up to be a distributor, and there is a small fee.

INDEX

Give the Gift of

He's Not Autistic, But...

How We Pulled Our Son From the Mouth of the Abyss

to Your Friends and Colleagues

CHECK YOUR LEADING BOOKSTORE OR ORDER HERE

❑ **YES**, I want _____ copies of *He's Not Autistic, But...* at $15.95 each, plus $4.95 shipping per book (Ohio residents please add $1.08 sales tax per book). Canadian orders must be accompanied by a postal money order in U.S. funds. Allow 15 days for delivery.

My check or money order for $_____ is enclosed.

Please charge my: ❑ Visa ❑ MasterCard

❑ Discover ❑ American Express

Name_____

Organization _____

Address _____

City/State/Zip _____

Phone_____ Email _____

Card # _____

Exp. Date_____ Signature _____

Please make your check payable and return to:

BookMasters, Inc.

30 Amberwood Parkway

Ashland, OH 44805

Call your credit card order to (800) 247-6553

Fax (419) 281-6883   order@bookmasters.com   www.atlasbooks.com

www.joyousmessenger.com